The Hemiplegia Handbook

The Hemiplegia Handbook for parents and professionals

by Liz Barnes and Charlie Fairhurst

2011
Mac Keith Press

© 2011 The Authors.

Editor: Hilary M Hart
Managing Director: Caroline Black
Production Manager: Udoka Ohuonu
Copy Editor: Gillian Whytock
Indexer: Pat Chappelle

First published in this edition 2011 by
Mac Keith Press, 6 Market Road, London N7 9PW, UK
Reprinted 2012.

British Library Cataloguing-in-Publication data.
A catalogue record of this book is available from the British Library.

ISBN: 978-1-907655-75-3

Typeset by Keystroke Typesetting and Graphic Design Ltd
Codsall, Wolverhampton
Printed by Latimer Trend & Company, Plymouth, Devon
Mac Keith Press is supported by Scope

Contents

About the authors

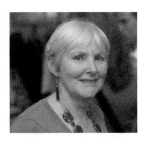

Liz Barnes is a trustee of HemiHelp and an award-winning radio journalist who for many years combined working for the BBC World Service with writing and editing much of HemiHelp's information material. She is a lay member of the National Institute for Health and Clinical Excellence (NICE) Guideline Development Group on Spasticity in Children and Young People. Liz lives in London with her husband and her son, now an adult, who was born with hemiplegia.

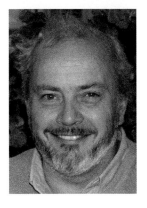

Dr Charlie Fairhurst is a consultant in paediatric neurodisability at the Evelina Children's Hospital in London where he is part of the South Thames regional movement therapy service. He has broad experience in helping families coping with acute and long-term neurological difficulties, especially the management of tone, posture, and function of the upper and lower limbs. He acts as a medical advisor for HemiHelp and sees children and young people with hemiplegia from throughout the UK to help with their clinical problems. He has published and presented on different areas of movement therapy, especially pain management and the importance of child- and family-based care.

Foreword

In 1990, when Carole Yude and I suggested to parents taking part in the London Hemiplegia Register that they might want to set up a new organization for children with hemiplegia and their families, we had no idea what this would lead to. Maybe no one would be interested. Maybe there would be a few poorly attended meetings before it all fizzled out. Instead, it all turned out far better than I could ever have dreamt. HemiHelp, as it became known has transformed the lives of thousands and done far more for children with hemiplegia than anything I could achieve as a doctor and researcher. I am a huge admirer of HemiHelp and everything that has grown out of it, including this marvellous handbook.

Written by a knowledgeable parent and a caring doctor, the book reflects what HemiHelp stands for. Everyone expects parents to be caring and doctors to be knowledgeable, but HemiHelp encourages us to be even more than this: empowering parents to be knowledgeable as well as caring, and helping doctors and other professionals to live up to their youthful ambition to be caring as well as knowledgeable. Of course, words are cheap, and any professional can say that they care. The real test is whether they are willing to go the extra mile – and no one can fault Charlie Fairhurst, who has gone many extra miles. Despite all the other demands on a consultant paediatrician, he has miraculously squeezed enough extra hours out of his day to share his vast knowledge and experience with us. Liz Barnes has given equally generously of her time, producing masterly chapters that bring together her professional skills as a journalist and her personal experience of what it is like to have a child with hemiplegia.

It is now common to talk of the importance of partnerships between parents and professionals, or between patients and professionals. Sometimes these are just empty words. Not so with HemiHelp, which has always been way ahead of the game. Long before this was fashionable, HemiHelp was organizing conferences so that professionals could help families and young people understand more about hemiplegia, and so that young people and families could help professionals understand what it was like to live with hemiplegia.

Families will treasure this handbook for many reasons. It shares practical tips and helps you realize that you are not alone. Other people have faced and overcome similar challenges, and their successes will help you find your own solutions. You may want to read the book from cover to cover, but I suspect that most of you will dip into it, starting with the parts that are relevant to your current circumstances. Next year's needs and interests will not be the same as today's, and you can turn to other parts of the book then.

At the risk of stating the obvious, it is perhaps worth saying that understanding more about the medical side of hemiplegia is not necessarily a walk in the park! Even with as good a guide as Charlie Fairhurst, it is an uphill road and it does require effort. Training as a medical student takes about five years, and becoming a specialist takes at least as long again. So don't be hard on yourself (or Charlie!) if you don't find it easy to understand everything on first reading. My advice is to skip over bits that seem too hard first time round and consider coming back to them later. You can't just walk straight up Everest.

If you are going to become a sort of medical student in order to make yourself more knowledgeable about hemiplegia, please see if you can avoid the medical student's fate of turning into a hypochondriac. Like so many of my fellow medical students, I would read about a new disease and all too readily start believing that I had those symptoms myself. You too may read in this book about rare complications and then start worrying that these will affect you or your child. Knowledge does not need to come at this price: forewarned and forearmed, I hope you will avoid needless anxiety.

Finally, I hope you enjoy this book as much as I have. It is a book that we have all been waiting for. I am sure you will agree that it was well worth the wait.

Robert Goodman
Institute of Psychiatry, London, UK

Chapter 1
Introduction

Liz Barnes

In the early 1990s, when he began his study of its causes and effects, Professor Robert Goodman described childhood hemiplegia as a 'Cinderella' condition. As recently as 2007 HemiHelp, the UK charity that provides support and information to people affected by the condition, had a letter from a man in his thirties who had only just discovered that he had hemiplegia while seeing his family doctor about something else. Even when it was diagnosed, hemiplegia was usually thought of as a mild physical disability, and families were left to get on with it with little or no support. And this was despite the fact that hemiplegia is quite a common condition, affecting about one child in a 1000.

Thankfully, things have moved on. Awareness of hemiplegia (also known as hemiparesis or hemiplegic cerebral palsy) in the medical professions has grown, and work by researchers around the world is adding to our knowledge of the condition. In particular, thanks to studies by Professor Goodman and others, people are much more aware that hemiplegia is not just a question of a weak arm and leg with, for some children, a few 'associated conditions', as they were referred to at the time, such as epilepsy, perhaps, or difficulties with some subjects at school. We now recognize it as a complex condition in which these hidden difficulties are not only more common than was realized previously but often have a more serious effect on the child's life than the more obvious ones. In other words, with hemiplegia what you see is not what you get. It is not surprising that parents, in the early years, and later on the young people themselves, find themselves constantly having to explain hemiplegia to the world at large.

But now at least they have rather more sources of information to refer to. In 1990 a handful of parents whose children had taken part in Professor Goodman's study set up HemiHelp as a support group to try to help others in the same situation. My son was too young to be included in the study, but I joined the group a year or so later. Since then I've been closely involved in writing and editing HemiHelp's information materials, which cover a wide range of practical issues from bikes to benefits and from shoelaces to Statements of Special Educational Needs. HemiHelp members tell us that they find these very helpful, especially now that they can be downloaded from the charity's website. However, I have felt for many years that it would be useful to have a book that would give a fuller picture of hemiplegia, its causes and effects and how to get on with living with it – whether you are a person with the condition, a family member, or a teacher or other professional working with children with hemiplegia. And now it has happened. This is in fact the second book on the subject to be published in the UK, but the first, *Congenital Hemiplegia,** is aimed at medical professionals and can be a hard read for anyone else.

Of course, no book can tell the reader everything, but my co-author, Dr Charlie Fairhurst, and I have tried to cover all the main areas. As part of the preparation for writing this handbook, HemiHelp carried out a survey of its parent members, and asked them, among other things, what they would like to see in it. About a quarter of parent members completed the survey, and from their answers it became clear that it was important for parents to know as much as possible about their child's condition, as the more they knew, the better prepared they would be to fight for the best possible help and support for him or her.

Each chapter of this handbook covers one subject, broken down into sections on different aspects and how they relate to children of different ages, from babies to teenagers and beyond. So parents, teachers and other professionals can dip into the handbook again and again as a child grows and their needs change. They will also find contact details for the many organizations that can provide more information, or help with complex matters such as applying for financial benefits or getting a Statement of Special Educational Needs. There are references, too, to information sheets, downloadable from the HemiHelp website (www.hemihelp.org.uk/hemiplegia/ publications/leaflets/), that cover individual topics in greater detail than there is space for here. And, since one of the most valuable things that people can have as they meet the challenges of living with hemiplegia is other people's personal experience, we have also included stories and suggestions from parents, as well as young people and adults who have grown up with the condition. Many thanks to all of them for their contribution, and to everyone who completed the survey as well as parents who sent us photographs to illustrate the book.

Most childhood hemiplegia is what is known as *congenital* (in other words, it developed before or around the time of the child's birth), so much of the handbook assumes that this is the kind of hemiplegia we are talking about. Of HemiHelp family members, 80% have a child whose condition is congenital; the other 20% have a child who 'acquired' his or her hemiplegia later in childhood as the result of an accident or illness, and we have included a section on *acquired hemiplegia*, as this is known (see Chapter 4). However, most of the information contained in the handbook is equally useful for both types.

Congenital Hemiplegia, eds Neville B, Goodman R. London: Mac Keith Press; 2001.

Although there are children with hemiplegia in every country, approaches to treatment and provision of services differ around the world, and for want of space we have had to aim this handbook mainly at readers in the UK. Even here, although health, social and education services are broadly similar throughout the UK, there are local differences in both how they are organized and what they are called, and we have tried to reflect this in the relevant chapters.

This handbook is also coming out at a time when significant changes are planned for the National Health Service, the benefits system and the support our children will receive during their education. So some of what is written here may be out of date before you read it. For this reason we have set up a dedicated page on the HemiHelp website for corrections and updates, and refer our readers to this in the relevant sections.

A word about labels: medical professionals use a number of names when they diagnose this condition: hemiplegia, hemiparesis, 'hemiplegic cerebral palsy' or sometimes just cerebral palsy. Many parents are unhappy about using this last name, especially if their child's hemiplegia seems mild. Others find it useful as a label because everyone has heard of it – I have sometimes said that my son has a sort of mild cerebral palsy, or talked about him having had a sort of stroke before he was born. Likewise, some parents are content to use the words 'disabled' and 'disability' when talking about their child, others not. Obviously this may depend on how mild or severe the hemiplegia seems. But, as parents, we can sometimes find ourselves using a word we would rather not use, either because it is easier to understand or because it seems useful at the time. When my son was diagnosed, his hemiplegia seemed fairly mild and mainly affected his arm, and when he went to a local mainstream playgroup I told just them that he had something called hemiplegia, which made his right arm and hand weak. Then, when he was about three and a half and ready for a primary school nursery class, I discovered that the school I had chosen had lost his application. The head teacher told me that they had no places left at nursery, and I knew that the same would be true of other local schools. I realized that I had one card up my sleeve, took a deep breath and said, 'Well actually he

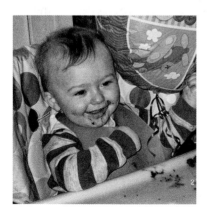

has a mild disability and I think he needs to have time in nursery to get used to the hustle and bustle of school before reception class.' I have never seen anyone's ears prick up like that before or since – within a week he had a place. Since then I have realized that, sometimes, if we want help for our children, we have to use whatever means we can, and it is difficult to avoid using labels such as 'disability' or 'cerebral palsy'. In the same way, a Statement of Special Educational Needs should be seen as an opportunity to get more help, not as a punishment. Remember that these are just labels and your child is always your child.

Bringing up any child is a voyage into the unknown – bringing up a child with a disability or additional needs even more so. The road ahead is less predictable, the challenges and obstacles greater, the anxieties deeper. But you need to remember that your child with hemiplegia is, first and foremost, a child like any other, and can grow up to lead a happy, useful adult life. We hope that this handbook will help you on your journey.

Note: All website information sheets, booklets etc., mentioned in this book are downloadable for free unless otherwise stated. References in this book to parents also apply to carers.

Chapter 2
Understanding the brain and movement

Charlie Fairhurst

I really wanted someone just to tell us, properly, why this had happened to our son. Not to pretend we knew too much or too little, just to tell us straight in a way we could understand . . .
Steve, Ashford

Some people may find this chapter rather daunting, especially if their child has only recently been diagnosed with hemiplegia. However, to truly understand how to manage a problem we have to start at the beginning. You may prefer to come back to this chapter later, particularly the parts to do with early brain development.

In medicine, when we start thinking about how to deal with a problem with the human body we work from our knowledge of the basic science of how it works normally. Doctors spend years at medical school learning about the development, anatomy and workings of the brain. All this knowledge becomes useful only when it is finally put into clinical practice. A good, basic understanding of how the hugely complex brain and nervous system works is the bedrock of neurological management. It guides sensible practice and is the core of proper communication, not only between members of the medical team but most importantly between professionals, children and their families.

So that we can truly understand how to help children with what is at basis a neurological problem, this chapter starts with a guide to how the brain develops and works. This will help us to understand more about what happens when a child is affected.

The development of the nervous system (see Figure 2.1)

Development of the brain
We all start off in basically the same way. From the moment of conception, cells start to double rapidly until a ball of cells is formed – a *morula*. This ball travels down the

fallopian tubes and starts to differentiate into an inner and outer core (a *blastocyst*), implanting itself into the lining of the womb about eight days after conception (all dates will be given as time after conception). The outer layer creates the placenta and membranes that a foetus needs for safe growth, and the inner ball of the blastocyst forms the *embryo*.

The ball starts to separate further into three layers, rather like a doughnut. The inner core (the jam or custard filling) is the *endoderm*, which goes on to make most of the organs of our body. The next layer (the dough) is the *mesoderm*, which makes the bones and muscles; and the outer layer (the deep-fried sugary coating) is the *neuro-ectoderm*, which makes the skin and nerves.

In the fourth week of development the ball begins to flatten out into a disc, keeping the three-layer system (like a squashed doughnut at the bottom of a shopping bag). One side of the outer neuro-ectoderm forms a *neural plate*, leaving the other side to create skin. This plate forms a *neural groove* down the middle and rolls up around itself into a tube – the *neural tube*, closing up along the back, up and down from the middle.

Soon afterwards the upper end of the neural tube gradually bends, flexes and wraps up on itself to form what is, by 11 weeks, a fairly recognizable brain-like structure, while the remainder becomes the spinal cord. From then on, specialization continues within the brain while development in the rest of the body catches up; the brain folds in on itself to form the convoluted surface, and new nerve cell (*neuron*) pathways and different supporting cell types continue to develop.

These pathways form from all parts of the brain down the spinal cord to all areas of the body, with restructuring, regression and organization into those seen in the mature brain occurring from around 24 weeks onwards.

When we are born the brain is more than 10% of our entire body weight, whereas by adulthood it is only 2%. At birth the brain is therefore comparatively large, but it does not stop developing. New cell types continue to be made, new nerve pathways come and go, the wiring of the nerve junctions becomes ever more complex, and myelin develops (fatty insulation of the electrical circuitry in the nervous system).

Because of all this, the brain that weighed about 350–400 grams at birth has increased to one kilogram by the time the baby is one year old, and by about two years of age its relative size, proportions and subdivisions are pretty similar to those of an adult. It is this massive growth of the brain after we are born that differentiates us from other mammals.

This period of rapid brain growth is a time of great risk for the development of neurological problems. Each structure in the nervous system has a period when it is particularly sensitive to the composition of the fluid surrounding the foetus in the developing womb. If constituents such as nutrients, growth factors and hormones are not present in the correct amounts at one of the critical points, or other things are present that should not be, then development can go wrong. One can see that it is a

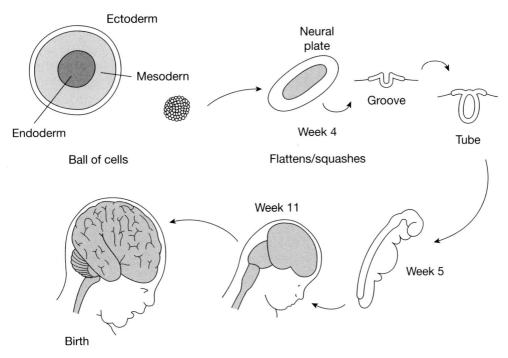

Figure 2.1. The development of the nervous system.

process fraught with the possibility of structures developing wrongly or pathways going haywire. Many of the earliest structural problems of the brain that lead on to congenital hemiplegia are the result of the development process going wrong.

Development of the blood supply to the brain
The development of the central nervous system is only half the problem, particularly in the context of this book. For the brain to function properly after birth, there needs to be an efficient way of getting energy, 'building blocks' and oxygen in and waste products out, i.e. an efficient blood supply is required. The development of the blood supply to the brain takes time and is fraught with its own risks.

The blood supply to the brain from the heart is split in two (See Figure 2.2). Half comes from the front of the head and flows back (through the *internal carotid arteries*), and half comes from the back of the head and flows forwards (through the *vertebral arteries*). In an embryo the development of the process to supply blood to the brain starts hand in hand with the development of the underlying structures of the brain, as outlined above. This begins towards the end of the first three months of pregnancy (the first trimester). However, at this stage the blood flow is poorly developed, and the foetus does not have the ability to keep things going independently of the mother's placenta until at least the middle of the second trimester (about 24 weeks). Even then, the immature and fragile blood supply can be disrupted for a whole host of reasons, mostly as a result of chance rather than specific medical associations.

The arteries of the brain start forming at the front and back of the surface of the brain, creeping towards the centre and burrowing deeper. Thus, the blood supply to the middle of the brain is not fully formed by the middle of pregnancy, so the areas most at risk from problems caused by a lack of oxygen or energy are likely to be deep within the brain. These areas include the motor pathways – the *corticospinal tracts* – which coordinate our movements by relaying messages from the brain motor cortex down to the spinal cord and from there to the musculoskeletal system.

Loss of this blood supply providing energy and oxygen to the motor pathways on one side of the brain is therefore an important cause of congenital hemiplegia. However, the longer that the foetus continues growing in the womb, the less likely the motor pathways are to be affected by fluctuations in blood flow and energy supply, as the placenta buffers the system so well.

When the baby is ready to be born (i.e. at full term) most of the brain, especially the *cortex* (the outer layer), is pretty robust and at less risk from changes in blood flow, oxygenation and energy supply. However, around this time the deepest parts of the brain – the *basal ganglia* – are so active and energy-consuming that they become prone to damage if starved of oxygen and energy for a relatively short period, say 10–15 minutes. These, as we shall see, are also areas that are vital in managing motor control and coordination.

The developed nervous system
The workings of the nervous system can seem very complicated, so I will not go into a mass of detail here but will explain the basics.

The central nervous system
The *central nervous system* consists of the brain at the top and the spinal cord sending messages downwards from the brain to control movement and upwards to the brain with information from our senses. From the central nervous system, messages pass to our muscles and from our senses along smaller nerves – the *peripheral nervous system*.

At the age of 18 years the brain weighs about 1.275 kilograms in women and 1.36 kg in men. The brain itself is subdivided into three main functional areas (some would say five but to keep things simple we will stick to three). On the top, covered in folds and convolutions, is the *cerebrum*. This is partially split into two *hemispheres* – left and right. Underneath it sits the *brainstem*, and behind this at the base of the brain is the *cerebellum*.

Each of the hemispheres is then divided into four lobes, named after the bones that overlie them: the frontal, parietal, temporal and occipital lobes. Each of these has specific roles to play in our senses, thoughts, words and deeds. For example, there is a well-defined *visual cortex* (responsible for processing what we see), a *sensory cortex* (responsible for processing what we feel by touch) and a *motor cortex* (responsible for coordinating our movements; see Figure 2.3), as well as areas responsible for speech and hearing. Although the areas of the brain associated with 'simple' movements and senses can be easily and accurately identified, when it comes to higher functioning, such as language, there is a greater degree of complexity and 'dominance' of one side of the brain over the other.

Towards the centre of each hemisphere is a fluid-filled space called a *ventricle*. Many of the long tracts that take messages from the cortex to the brainstem and beyond are situated around the ventricles – in the *periventricular* area. Each hemisphere interacts primarily with the opposite side of the body, messages about movements crossing at the brainstem level. It also interacts with the other hemisphere through a large bundle of nerves, the *corpus callosum*, which connects the mirror image points of each hemisphere.

The brainstem is a hugely complicated network of groups of cells, such as the basal ganglia, and pathways, not unlike an old-fashioned telephone exchange. Most of our automatic feelings, emotions and movements rely on this area working properly.

The brain needs about one-fifth of the blood supply, oxygen and energy requirements of the whole body. This makes it pretty greedy, given its comparatively small size in adults. The blood flows up to the brain through the pair of frontal internal carotid arteries and the pair of back vertebral arteries. These form a loop at the base of the brain from which a number of arteries branch off (see Figure 2.2). The most important of these, for our purposes, is the one most frequently affected by a blockage arising from damage, a blood clot or a small amount of the fluid that surrounds the foetus (an *amniotic embolus*) entering the artery – the middle cerebral artery. This artery feeds and oxygenates the basal ganglia and motor areas of the cortex and takes away the waste products.

The peripheral motor system
To control movement, messages are transmitted by the central nervous system from the spinal cord out to the groups of muscles that work as a *motor unit*, contracting and relaxing in order to move our skeleton. (Muscles work in pairs at each joint: an *agonist* muscle, or the chunkier of the pair, e.g. the biceps at the elbow, and an *antagonist* muscle, the feebler of the pair, e.g. the triceps at the elbow.)

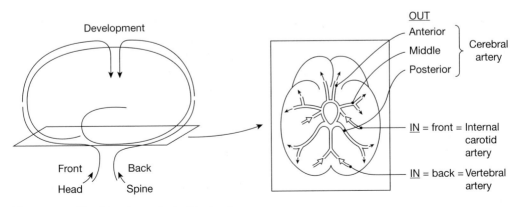

Figure 2.2. The blood supply to the brain.

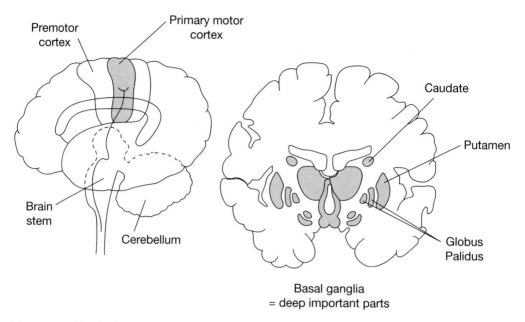

Premotor cortex

Primary motor cortex

Caudate

Putamen

Brain stem

Cerebellum

Globus Palidus

Basal ganglia = deep important parts

Figure 2.3. The brain.

Messages about the world around us are also relayed from our hands, arms, feet, legs, and so on, using all our different senses, back to the spinal cord and upwards to the brain. These messages are relayed by peripheral nerves: these can be thought of as simple wiring to and from the central nervous system, going in from the senses or out to the motor unit. Simple chemical transmitters are used to pass information across the small gaps or *synapses* between the various elements of these systems: for example, from the central corticospinal pathway to the peripheral motor nerve and then on to the muscles.

I hope from this description of how the brain and nervous system work together that it is clear how a localized brain injury, or *impairment*, caused for example by a lack of blood flow, will lead to specific functional difficulties or *disabilities* for the person concerned. The specific patterns of functional clinical difficulties can almost always be traced back to the part of the brain that has not developed normally or has sustained injury.

This knowledge of what happens in the normal and abnormal brain is the basis of all our clinical practice in helping people with hemiplegia.

Movement – when it works

Background
Motor control is the way that the brain and nervous system direct our muscles to move or carry out actions. As far as motor control is concerned, our brains are basically very

similar to those of the catfish, except that we have a large cortex on top. A catfish swims rhythmically through murky waters, opening its mouth and sucking in everything that goes past. It does not worry about the weather or what to wear or even how to scratch that itch: all those worries come from the greater development of our brain that happened at a later evolutionary stage. We and the catfish do, however, have a similar basic nervous system drive for movement, the *locomotor driving system* (see Figure 2.4). This functional area of the brain controls what goes on at the spinal level – the *central pattern generators* – where patterns of movements are organized by different groups of muscles. Simple *motor pattern generation* (the way in which nerves generate motor commands for muscles to carry out movements such as walking) follows the same basic system in all creatures with nerves, bones and muscles.

Humans have a complicated multilevel system of muscles that work to move the skeleton in different directions by contracting and relaxing across joints, but the same principles apply. The coordination of this system is vital in order to develop skills of normal posture and movement.

Normal posture and movement
We all know from watching babies that the patterns of movement in early development are similar in almost everybody. We tend to sit before we crawl, crawl before we stand, and stand before we walk. These skills are synchronized by patterns in the physical development of the nervous system.

Even in the womb the spinal cord coordinates a wide variety of *motor reflexes*: simple rhythmic movements of different muscles that we can perform without thinking. When we are born, these primitive reflexes can be seen in the *patterns* involved in rooting for the nipple, sucking and swallowing. As our brains grow, similar yet increasingly complex motor unit patterns develop related to the functioning of our body, limbs and trunk.

These rhythmic motor patterns initiated in the spinal cord – the central pattern generators – have to be started, directed, speeded up and slowed down. We do this by using the central nervous system to switch on and off the motor nerves that in turn control the muscles working together in the motor unit. It is the deepest parts of the brain (or basal ganglia) that manage this basic turning on and off of signals – this is the *locomotor driving system*.

On top of this, as thinking, learning and communicating beings, we have ways of using all the other input from sight, sound, temperature, touch, pain, balance and position senses to adapt the way we move – this is the *cortical adaptive system*. As well as this adaptive section, other parts of the brain are important in using input messages to keep us balanced and upright, for example the cerebellum – this is the *equilibrium system*. These higher-functioning areas of our brain interact and fiddle with the output of the locomotor driving messages sent down from the brainstem to the spinal levels, helping us change the direction and speed of movement.

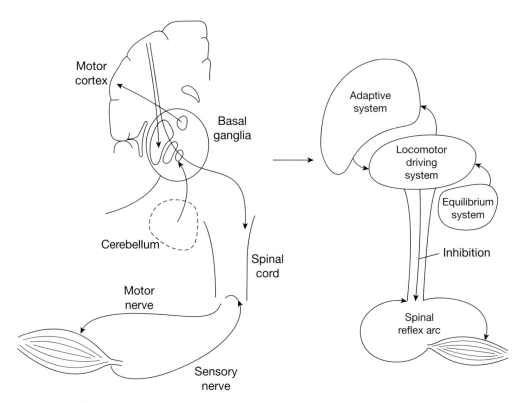

Figure 2.4. The control of movement.

At the spinal and peripheral nerve level there occurs what we call the spinal reflex arc. This is the basic information loop that causes the knee to jump when the doctor hits it with a tendon hammer. The peripheral receptor in the tendon tells the spinal cord that it is being stretched, which in turns fires off the motor unit that is connected to that specific tendon. Normally the brain then acts rapidly to chill out the system – *descending inhibition*. Without normal descending motor control the motor unit continues to fire and hence function and ability are lost. This is what happens in a central movement disorder such as hemiplegia.

I hope I have now explained the basics of how the brain and central nervous system coordinate our movements. However, in order to make movement happen we need an integrated skeletal system of bones and joints, with muscles and tendons overlying them to act as the power packs and ropes (*peripheral motor unit*). In children even this simple-sounding biomechanical system is complicated. Bone growth is largely under hormonal control. Growth and (at puberty) sex hormones stimulate special *growth plates* at the top and bottom of our bones, where cells divide and the bones become longer.

Muscles and tendons, on the other hand, grow because physical forces stimulate their growth plate, the point where muscles and tendons come together. Therefore, if the muscle does not stretch and relax efficiently, as is the case when the brain is not controlling it normally, then the muscle will tighten up more quickly and joint movements become increasingly limited, as happens when young people grow older.

Movement – when it doesn't work

When there is disruption of all these interacting links, the system cannot function properly: there is a structural impairment. A great deal of research has been done on how much *plasticity* there is in the central nervous system, once damage has occurred, to minimize the potential disability. The concept of plasticity is that the brain has a built-in ability to relearn or rewire after being damaged. It has been proved that the brain can do this, at least to some extent. However, how we can best make use of this potential is unclear. We will go into much greater detail when we look at interventions in Chapter 6. In the meantime, we suggest that you keep an open mind on this concept.

In spite of this potential to rewire, at the visible level the brain does not regrow after damage. Clinicians can learn a lot from images of the brain (e.g. with MRI). Having said that, many of the children I see with the most profound difficulties have near-normal brain scans, and others with very mild disabilities have brains that show areas of severe damage. Again, we will focus on the basics of our understanding of what goes wrong.

We have covered together how we initiate and control our movement. When irreversible damage occurs in the central nervous system, it can affect some or all of the descending pathways coordinating our movement. This can lead to a change in motor control and muscle activity – the so-called *upper motor neuron syndrome*. This is a complex pattern of movement difficulties with a range of 'positive' and 'negative' features, the balance of which affects each person's level of functional disability. In normal speech positive = good and negative = bad, whereas with hemiplegia this may not be the case.

The 'positive' features come from the lack of descending inhibition, which leads to muscle groups being overactivated. This creates two clinical difficulties. The first is *spasticity*; the second comes from all the muscles firing off in an uncontrolled pattern.

Most of us will have heard of spasticity but few, including most doctors, understand exactly what it means. When the peripheral motor unit is constantly overfiring, as the brain cannot switch it off, the muscle property (its structure and how it behaves) changes dramatically. Those spinal reflexes fire off without control (*hyper-reflexia*), the *tone* (tension) of the muscle increases (*hypertonia*), the muscles become very twitchy (*clonus*), and all muscles normally coordinated by a particular spinal level fire off together (*co-contraction*). This in turn leads to the mass activation of muscles in abnormal patterns.

This is a big problem in its own right, but, when spasticity causes changes in the properties of the muscle, then how it can work becomes even more limited. Constant overactivation of the peripheral motor unit causes changes in the make-up of the muscles and the length of the muscle–tendon complexes. The muscles become full of connective tissue, rather than muscle fibres, and the nature of the remaining fibres changes so that they become much more sluggish. As we discussed above, over time there is a relative slowing of growth, so that the muscles and tendons become 'tighter' – *contractures* are formed. This tightness has generally been the focus for most treatment of spasticity (physiotherapy, occupational therapy and surgery).

The flip side to this tightness is the 'negative' factor of the upper motor neuron syndrome. As well as the overactivation of muscle groups, there is a contrary reduction in motor activity leading to three outcomes: a loss in dexterity (clumsiness); a loss in selective motor control (ability to coordinate movements); and muscle weakness. These three factors can be just as disabling for the person concerned as the 'tightness', if not more so, but generally receive less attention.

More than just a movement problem

As we explained above, problems can occur at any point of foetal, infant, child or adult growth and development. Although we have so far focused on movement, it is vitally important to remember that the system is far more complex.

There is careful interrelation of the neural pathways coordinating our special senses – thinking, feeling and emotions – especially in the deep parts of the brain. Communication and understanding are also primarily dealt with in specific areas, some of which are closely related to the motor cortex, especially on the left side of the brain. A problem that initially shows up as a movement disorder is likely also to cause difficulties in many of these other areas. We will go through this in more detail in Chapter 4, using the concepts of how all the parts of the nervous system work together to explain the difficulties associated with hemiplegia.

Summary
- Brain growth is complicated.
- A lot can go wrong with the brain structurally during all stages of development as a result of fluctuations in blood and energy supply.
- Movement is controlled by the interaction of the central nervous system and the peripheral motor unit.
- Some parts of the brain are particularly important in motor control; these are often the areas most susceptible to damage as we grow inside and outside the womb.

- When impairment in the central nervous system happens, an imbalance in muscle tightness and weakness occurs, causing disability.
- A child grows rapidly: if there is an underlying problem in movement, subsequent imbalance in growth makes things even more complicated.
- Bones grow in response to hormones. Muscles and tendons grow as a result of mechanical stimulus and need normal patterns of movement to keep up with the underlying bone growth.
- A structural problem with growth and development in half of the brain is unlikely to lead to a movement disorder alone. Many children with hemiplegia and their families find that other elements of their neurological condition, such as behavioural issues and epilepsy, create far more problems.

Chapter 3
Causes of hemiplegia/ hemiparesis

Charlie Fairhurst

I spent ages going over his pregnancy in my mind. Was there anything I did wrong, anything I could have done different. It must have been my fault, I was certain, I was his mum . . .

Debbie, Hastings

The aim of the last chapter was to explain how the brain develops and works and to introduce some of the ways in which things can go wrong. For professionals, that is the basis of appreciating why problems occur and working out how to help. We will now focus on what happens specifically in hemiplegia, looking at the stages of foetal or childhood development at which the problems may occur.

Some terms and definitions

It is probably easiest to start by giving a few important medical definitions, followed by a description of the effects of a unilateral brain problem, and then some tables describing what can cause a hemiplegic movement disorder.

> **Congenital** This means present at or before birth, or soon after birth, although the signs may not become obvious until much later.
>
> **Acquired** This means arising or occurring later.
>
> **Cerebral palsy** This is 'a group of disorders of motor function, movement and posture; it is "permanent but not unchanging" and is caused by non-progressive lesions [injuries] or abnormalities in the developing/immature brain (up to about 18–24 months of age).' This means that, even though the impairment of the brain is static, because we are growing beings, the problems encountered change and can develop over time. It is important to stress that this is a description and not a specific diagnosis, even though this is an extremely common medical label.

If you use the term **'hemiplegic or unilateral cerebral palsy'**, possible causes can be both congenital or early acquired (up to 18-24 months of age).

> **Hemiplegia** [Greek: 'hemi' = half, 'plegia' = loss of function] Specifically in medical texts, this is defined as 'a one-sided pattern of muscle overactivation and reduction in motor activity, leading to increased muscle tightness, and reflexes, weakness and loss of selective motor control'.

> **Hemiparesis** [Greek: 'hemi' = half, 'paresis'= weakness] On the other hand this is defined as 'a partial paralysis with incomplete loss of muscle power on one side of the body'.

Understandably the terms 'hemiplegia' and 'hemiparesis' are frequently used as if they were the same by professionals; here in the United Kingdom, many of the great tomes of paediatric neurology interchange the two terms as if they were one and the same. However, other parts of the world either tend to favour one term or the other (in the USA, for example, 'hemiparesis' is the preferred term), or use them to make a distinction between a more serious condition ('hemiplegia') and a milder one ('hemiparesis'). Basically they are both used to describe a movement disorder involving one half of the body. However, it is rare not to have some subtle neurological difficulties on the opposite (contralateral) side of the body too.

> **Spasticity/hypertonia** This is a problem with movement associated with damage to the adaptive motor system (see Chapter 2), i.e. the motor cortex to corticospinal tracts, that leads in turn to increased muscle tone and reflexes, and problems with all muscles firing off – *co-contraction*. This 'high muscle tone' happens because an abnormal descending motor control does not switch off the firing of the muscles.

> **Dyskinesis/dystonia** This is a problem of the central nervous system associated with the basal ganglia not working properly – the locomotor driving system (see Chapter 2) – leading to a loss of fluidity in movement. There is generally a fluctuating muscle tone pattern – from tight when stressed, anxious or tired to relatively good functional ability when relaxed. The muscles are generally relaxed at night time.

It is rare to see a movement disorder that is completely one or the other of these two patterns (hypertonia, dystonia). Generally one dominates (usually hypertonia), depending on whether the main structural problem of the brain is in the cortex (hypertonia) or the basal ganglia (dystonia).

There are more subtle breakdowns of the different patterns of movement, and you may come across terms such as chorea, athetosis, and so on. However, for our purposes, it is easier and entirely reasonable to stick with the concepts of high, low and fluctuating muscle tone – hypertonia, hypotonia and dystonia, respectively.

The following are definitions of some of the most common terms used in the diagnosis of hemiplegia.

Intraventricular haemorrhage (IVH) Bleeding into the fluid-filled space in the centre of the cerebral hemisphere (where the blood vessels are most fragile).

Periventricular haemorrhagic infarction (PHI) Tissue damage caused by bleeding into the areas of the brain closest to the edge of the internal ventricles. Often seen in babies after a premature delivery as, once again, these are the areas where the blood vessels are most susceptible to damage from low oxygen or fluctuation in blood pressure.

Periventricular leukomalacia (PVL) Damage to the cells and central nervous system pathways close to the ventricle on the inside of the brain, following an intraventricular haemorrhage or a periventricular haemorrhagic infarction.

Hypoxic ischaemic encephalopathy (HIE) [Hypoxic = low oxygen, ischaemic = lack of blood flow, encephalopathy = damage to the brain] This is damage to the brain caused by loss of blood flow and oxygen. It is generally found in infants that have a profound difficulty at or around the time of labour, for example from a loss of placental blood flow (caused by abruption – the placenta coming away from the womb lining – or cord prolapse – when the umbilical cord precedes the baby during birth) or if the birth is difficult.

At the end of the book is a glossary of medical terms.

Congenital causes of hemiplegia

Obviously, it is important for the medical world to know how common movement disorders are as a whole in children and young people. Over the years, there has been a great deal of research into congenital hemiplegia. One of the largest studies has been the European Collaborative Study, published in 2007, which involved 16 centres across Europe. Because of the lag times involved in such large studies, its results concern the incidence of all types of cerebral palsy from 1980 to 2000 (including congenital and early acquired hemiplegia).

If we break the study findings down to look at causes present at or before birth, it shows that, unlike other movement disorders, the rate of congenital hemiplegia has not altered much over the 25 years up to 2010, remaining at just under one child per 1000. Other studies from the UK, Canada and Australia have shown similar results. For reasons generally related to blood flow to the brain while the baby is in the womb (intrauterine causes), right-sided hemiplegia continues to be slightly more common than left sided.

Table 3.1. Congenital causes of hemiplegia from conception to birth

When it happens	What happens	Examples
Conception	Genetic	All forms are rare The most common include tuberous sclerosis (a genetic disease causing a range of symptoms including seizures and developmental delay) and Sturge–Weber syndrome (a rare neurological and skin disorder)
	'Inborn errors of metabolism'	Mitochondrial disorders (within the cells) Peroxisomal (enzyme) disorders
Early pregnancy	Unilateral problems of brain development	Developmental cortical abnormalities Hemi – half + brain (cephalos) – hemicephaly Too little development – microcephaly Too much development – megalencephaly Wrong cells in wrong places – 'migration disorders' Brain 'organization disorders'
	Intrauterine infection (infection crossing from mother to foetus in the womb)	Toxoplasmosis, rubella, cytomegalovirus, herpesvirus (collectively known as TORCH) or many other viral infections
Mid-pregnancy	Blockage of blood supply to one half of brain – middle cerebral artery	Small amount of fluid surrounding foetus leaks into placental blood flow – embolus Blood clotting too easy (thrombophilia) Cause usually uncertain
	Failure of foetus to grow	Poor placental function
	Haemorrhage (bleed) into brain tissue	Intraventricular haemorrhage (IVH)
Later pregnancy but premature delivery	Haemorrhage into brain tissue Lack of oxygenation Reduced blood pressure Infections	Reduced blood pressure, reduced oxygenation of blood or damage from infection, leading to damage of blood vessels and periventricular haemorrhagic (PVH) infarctions in turn leading to periventricular leuckomalacia (PVL).
Late pregnancy (around the time of full-term delivery)	Haemorrhage into brain tissue Lack of oxygen/blood flow to the brain Infection	Maternal high blood pressure – 'eclampsia' Placental dysfunction/bleeding Hypoxic ischaemic encephalopathy (HIE) Mother – high fever Premature rupture of membranes Baby – bacterial septicaemia (blood poisoning)/meningitis (inflammation of the membranes covering the brain)

When does congenital hemiplegia arise?

Conception Taking the cause of a disorder from the earliest point of conception, problems associated with the genetic coding of how the central nervous system develops are rarely the only cause. There are, however, several specific 'syndromes' that have a pattern of clinical difficulties that include a hemiplegic movement disorder (see Table 3.1).

Early pregnancy Problems with the development of the brain in the very early stages of foetal development – the initial folding and moulding of the brain and subsequent development of neural pathways – are the cause of 5–15% of all cases of congenital hemiplegia. With regards to this, words you may recognize from medical language are such things as *schizencephaly* (smooth brain surface) and *pachygyria* (too few folds in the brain surface).

Mid–pregnancy Around 40–50% of all cases of congenital hemiplegia are caused by damage to an immature blood vessel or by a blocked blood vessel, usually the middle cerebral artery, when the baby is growing in the womb. These generally occur about the middle third (second trimester) of pregnancy. This haemorrhage, or *infarction*, leads to the classic *periventricular leuckomalacia* (PVL), whereby the pathways within the brain do not develop because of the damage incurred. Doctors often look for risk factors that may have led to damage of the immature blood vessels, such as an inborn increased risk of blood clotting or high maternal blood pressure (*pre-eclampsia/eclampsia*), but generally there is no specific reason and it is not related to anything occurring during the pregnancy, e.g. falling off your bicycle.

Late pregnancy/birth Birth is the next major risk factor, again causing about 10–20% of the total cases of congenital hemiplegia. Problems in a complicated delivery or prolonged labour are generally due to either a direct loss of blood flow (and therefore shortage of oxygen) to areas of the brain or clots and haemorrhages, as outlined above.

Prematurity

Extremely premature delivery (before 28 weeks) is obviously a major risk factor: although the number of children born this early is low, it still accounts for about 20% of children with congenital hemiplegia. The brain itself is fragile and, as we have shown in the last chapter, the blood supply is delicate and susceptible to clots and haemorrhages.

Within this prematurely born group, the European Collaborative Study on Cerebral Palsy showed that, when one looks at risk rates for *bilateral* movement disorders, there is a strong connection to the size of the baby. When born prematurely, the 'very low birthweight' infants have up to four to six times the relative risk of developing a movement disorder. Interestingly, this is not the same in a *unilateral* disorder (hemiplegia), where the risk rates are the same for premature infants less than 1 kilogram in weight as they are for those 1–1.5 kilograms, both being approximately 1% of each group.

Infection
Much more rarely, hemiplegia can be caused by an infection whilst the baby is growing in the womb. Such infections can cause damage at any stage of foetal development. It is important, however, to stress that this is rare (less than 5% of proven cases) and generally women should not worry about common viruses (e.g. colds or diarrhoea) that they catch when pregnant.

Early on, the so-called TORCH congenital infections (toxoplasmosis, rubella, cytomegalovirus, herpesvirus; see Table 3.1) can interfere with the normal development of the brain.

Later on in foetal development, severe maternal blood-borne bacterial infections (*septicaemia*) can lead to fluctuations in the rate of blood flow to the baby's brain. Very rarely (in fewer than 1% of proven cases), severe maternal infection can also directly interfere with the flow of blood in the placenta, thereby affecting the baby's circulatory system, leading to irreversible damage in the central nervous system. Near or at the time of delivery, infections of the womb can lead to meningitis or septicaemia in the baby, causing a direct effect on the brain.

After birth
Environmental and infective factors continue to pose a risk for the rapidly developing brain after the baby is born. Early meningitis in particular is a significant risk factor, as are emergency interventions by doctors to stabilize an otherwise sick baby that can cause clots and haemorrhages in the middle cerebral arteries (e.g. dialysis for babies with kidney failure or emergency surgical interventions for babies born with abnormal hearts or intestines).

Other possible risks
In any foetus growing in the womb there are a number of other risk factors that increase the likelihood of developing hemiplegia, apart from all those listed above. Obviously there is a lot of interest over whether other 'foetal environmental' factors, such as medicines, foods, drinks, drugs, direct trauma (physical injury), dental amalgam or coughs and colds, can lead to an increased relative risk. However, no direct link has been proven.

As specialists in this area we have come across rare cases of serious direct trauma, in which a unilateral brain abnormality can be shown subsequently in the growing foetus with ultrasound or neuroimaging, but these are very exceptional. Equally, some other viral infections, as well as medicines and drugs, can lead to problems in the development of the brain, but none are linked specifically to hemiplegia.

Medical science does not have all the answers. We live in a world that is not black and white but is composed of grey statistical probabilities. All I can tell you is that in huge epidemiological (causation) studies across the world over the last 50 years, nothing specific has come to light in many of these areas. Although we should not rule out anything, it is not helpful to look for specific answers that really are not there.

Twin and multiple pregnancies

As is clear, there are a large number of possible causes of congenital hemiplegia. The number of children being born with hemiplegia has not altered over the last 30 years, at around one in 1000, in spite of massive changes in obstetric and neonatal practice. Improvements in care are mirrored by increased rates of survival of very premature babies and multiple births from assisted conception. As the risk of any pregnancy and delivery increases with the number of babies in the womb, there is a slightly increased risk of congenital hemiplegia in twin pregnancies, which increases further with triplets and quadruplets.

Acquired causes of hemiplegia

In the HemiHelp survey of its members, fewer than one in five children had an acquired hemiplegia. Damage to the structures on one side of the brain after birth can be caused by many things, all of which are individually very rare indeed.

Acquired problems of the brain can occur at any age and stage of development from birth to old age. In childhood the vast majority of cases occur in the first three years of life. The onset of signs is generally very acute and severe, followed by a variable degree of recovery, depending on the underlying cause. We will cover this more fully in the next chapter.

When we doctors think about causes, we use a simple process of elimination called a 'surgical sieve'. We decide whether the cause is static or progressive in its pattern, and then whether it is vascular, infective, immune, metabolic, inflammatory, traumatic, epileptic or neoplastic (caused by a tumour) in origin.

I do not intend to go over the examples given above in detail – as stated, they are all very rare indeed – but I will give an idea why problems occur, breaking them down into the three areas of static (unchanging), progressive (worsening) and fluctuating difficulties. Much of what we have already covered in the section on congenital causes is equally relevant in the acquired.

Acquired static problems of the brain

Static causes can be vascular, infective, post-infective (a reactive process after an infection) or lesion- or trauma-related in origin.

> **Vascular** Blockage of blood vessels and haemorrhages can lead to damage to the nerves and pathways of the brain. The reasons for this can be multiple, and we look for clotting problems or causes of *thrombi* (clots, plural of *thrombus*) in the circulatory system (blood vessels and heart).
>
> **Infective** Meningitis or encephalitis (infection of the lining of the brain – the *meninges* – or the brain itself) can cause problems directly to brain cells and

Table 3.2. Acquired causes of hemiplegia

Type	Cause	Examples
Static problem of the brain	Blood vessel (vascular)	Right middle cerebral artery embolus and clot (thrombus) leading to infarction (cell death)
	Infective	Intracranial abscess Meningitis Bacterial Viral Encephalitis (inflammation of the brain) Chicken pox
	Post infective	Post rubella Post measles – subacute sclerosing panencephalitis (a rare type of chronic progressive encephalitis) Post-mumps encephalitis Rasmussen syndrome (another rare form of chronic encephalitis)
	Lesions	Neurocutaneous syndromes (i.e. affecting skin and nervous system; these are really congenital but they may not present until later) e.g. neurofibromatosis, tuberous sclerosis, Sturge–Weber syndrome Traumatic head injury
Progressive problem of the brain	Loss of cells – demyelinating disease	Relapsing–remitting multiple sclerosis
	Inflammation of blood vessels	Systemic lupus erythematosus (SLE) Henoch–Schönlein purpura (HSP)
	Recurrent 'mini-strokes'	Heart valve disease Coagulopathies (diseases affecting blood clotting) and platelet disorders Thrombotic (too much clotting, forming a thrombus), e.g. sickle cell disease, factor XII deficiency
	Lesions	Neoplasms – tumours (e.g. gliomas of brainstem, basal ganglia)
Fluctuating problem of the brain	Migrainous	Hemiplegic migraine
	Epilepsy	Post convulsive hemiplegia (after seizures) Hemiconvulsion–hemiplegia (unilateral 'status epilepticus')
	Vascular	Diabetes mellitus

pathways, or indirectly to the brain by damaging supplying blood vessels. Infection may also lead to abscess formation in the brain, whereby direct pressure causes damage to the brain.

Post-infective Some infections lead in turn to 'post-infective' states. These are rare, even in a world of rarity, and to develop hemiplegia rather than another neurological complication is almost unknown! Certain viral infections, such as measles, can cause a reaction in the brain that tricks our immune system into thinking that the brain is an infecting agent and therefore our own immune system starts attacking the brain, i.e. an autoimmune disorder.

There is huge parental anxiety over whether childhood immunization is a risk factor. Neurological complications of immunizations are uncommon, far more uncommon than the virus infection that they are preventing. Serious complications are extremely rare: in fact, in large-scale trials none of the childhood immunizations used in the UK, Europe, Australasia or the Americas have shown any epidemiological link to development of hemiplegia.

Lesions or growths Though they may be termed 'congenital' in origin, some genetic disorders become obvious only with time. These include the group called *neurocutaneous* disorders. As you will remember from the last chapter, the skin and nervous system are made from the same early foetal building blocks – the neuro-ectoderm. Some examples are given in the table above: the problems associated with hemiplegia arise if there is a benign growth or blood flow abnormality interfering with the motor pathways of the brain on one side.

Trauma All the following numbers are basically to put the area of head injuries into context, even though trauma is a comparatively common cause of an acquired hemiplegia:

- 10% of all children attending accident and emergency departments have suffered head trauma. The total incidence is around 290 per 100,000 children each year.
- 5–10% of these have a severe injury – 15–29 per 100,000 children per year.
- 20% of children with a severe head injury will also be left with a significant motor disability – approximately 4.5 per 100,000 children per year.
- About one-third of these will have a hemiplegic rather than a bilateral movement disorder.
- Therefore, the total incidence of acquired hemiplegia from significant head trauma is 1.5 per 100,000 children each year.

Having said all that, statistics are meaningless if you are among the 1.5 children or their families.

Severe accidental head injuries are mainly caused by road traffic accidents and falling from heights. Those causing hemiplegia are most commonly linked to penetrating injuries of the skull, fractures of the skull and bleeding into the brain (intracranial haemorrhages). We will talk about this in more detail in the next chapter.

Acquired progressive problems of the brain
Rarely, brain inflammation, the loss of cells or myelin (the fatty insulation of the nerve fibres) or growths that increase in size cause progressive damage to the brain. In children the most common of these rare conditions are degenerative problems of the brain and tumours of the brainstem, basal ganglia or thalamus (the base structures of the brain). Examples are given in Table 3.2 above.

Many diseases of the blood system, including stickiness of the platelets, too much or too little clotting or sickle cell disease (characterized by 'sickle-shaped' red blood cells that can block blood vessels) can lead to recurrent 'mini-strokes', as can *emboli* (any foreign material in the blood capable of obstructing the blood vessel, plural of *embolus*) originating in the heart. These can show up as a progressive problem in the pathways of the brain more frequently than a static problem.

Acquired fluctuating problems of the brain
Migraine and epilepsy can lead to a fluctuating loss of movement on one side of the body

> **Hemiplegic migraine** is another rare condition that is usually genetic in origin, running in families. Loss of speech and motor (movement) function is associated with spasms of the blood vessels in the brain. Genetic investigations should be done – but nothing causing too much trauma as that might provoke the spasms.

> More frequently, in other migrainous problems there may be a more **transient loss of movement** in the *aura* phase (an early stage of neurological disturbance before the onset of headache associated with some types of migraine, in which the sufferer experiences disturbances of perception).

> Another extremely rare condition, known as **alternating hemiplegia of childhood**, almost always begins in the first year of life. There is generally fluctuating stiffness and discomfort with a wide variety of neurological presentation. The side involved alternates.

> **Prolonged epileptic seizures** can lead to hemiplegia if only one side of the brain is involved.

> There is also a **post-convulsive hemiplegia,** where movement returns after a period of minutes to hours.

> **Acute, transitory attacks of hemiplegia** can occur in children with insulin-dependent diabetes. These episodes usually occur when the child is sleeping and may last for hours, but the child will recover fully.

Summary

- 'Hemiplegia' and 'hemiparesis' are terms often used interchangeably in the UK.

- Hemiplegia can be either congenital or acquired:
  - 'congenital' means that the brain damage that caused the hemiplegia happened before or at around the time of birth;
  - 'acquired' means that the hemiplegia is a result of injury or illness during childhood.

- There are many different causes of hemiplegia. The most common are these:
  - problems with brain development;
  - problems with blood flow to the brain;
  - infections and inflammation of the brain; and
  - trauma to the brain or blood vessels.

Chapter 4

Possible clinical problems: their signs and symptoms

Charlie Fairhurst

We were first-time parents; we didn't understand that there was anything wrong; our health visitor and GP just told us it was because Tom was born too early.

Andrew, Bath

Our expectation was that we were going to manage with a physically disabled child but that his learning would be normal. As time goes by he is managing physically very well but the learning things seem to be falling behind.

Ranjini, Birmingham

We humans cannot run across the savannah minutes after we are born in order to escape a hungry predator. The long and complex brain development described in previous chapters means that eventually, however, we may be able to understand advanced astrophysics, play football for Manchester United, or even be a contestant on the X Factor. But we all start out as wriggling, dependent babies.

The normal pattern of human motor development means that an infant should lie symmetrically by a few months, sit independently by eight months, stand at around one year and walk before 18 months of age. Children with hemiplegia usually reach these milestones at a similar age, unless their motor impairment is very severe. However, the pattern of movements seen will be different from those of a typically developing child.

In Chapter 2 we saw what happens when the motor system works, and what happens when it goes wrong. The damaged areas of the brain fail to coordinate muscles, and this can show as weakness or tightness, loss of dexterity, or problems with selective motor control. More rarely the child will have an abnormal pattern of fluctuating movement – a 'dys-' (abnormal) 'kinesis' (movement).

Congenital hemiplegia

Congenital hemiplegia is rarely picked up at birth, unless an antenatal ultrasound scan shows either a structural abnormality of the brain or an abnormality arising from thrombosis (obstruction of a blood vessel by a clot). In a very young baby the nervous system is not sufficiently mature for any one-sidedness to be obvious. Therefore, only about one in ten children are clinically diagnosed by four to five months and only half by ten months of age.

If a movement problem on one side is seen in a very young baby, it is not normally associated with damage to the brain but rather to the nerves travelling in the shoulder and arm after they have left the spinal cord – the *brachial plexus*. Damage to these nerves is not a hemiplegia but a *palsy*, generally the result of birth trauma – the nerves being excessively stretched during a difficult birth. The arm is floppy and has no reflexes present and the leg is not affected at all. This is the most common early misdiagnosis.

Obviously, if your baby has been in the special-care baby unit, you may already be aware of structural problems with one side of the brain. During their time on such units most babies have regular check-up ultrasound scans of the head that pick up haemorrhages in the ventricles or into the matter of the brain itself. As stated in Chapter 3, we know that the risk factors are many, and medical teams will probably pick up possible structural brain damage, using diagnostic imaging techniques such as cranial ultrasound or magnetic resonance imaging (MRI).

However, most children do not have a premature delivery, an abnormal antenatal scan or a difficult birth. In these, the most common way of diagnosing hemiplegia is that one arm or hand 'seems to be working better' at an early stage. Normally children do not have any degree of left- or right-handedness before the age of 18–24 months. Therefore, if a child is using only one hand for most early tasks of reaching and exploring, it is not because he or she is developmentally advanced, but because the other side has a problem with motor control – weakness, selectivity (ability to make fluid movements) and stretchable tightness. It may be that the hand is held in a 'fisted posture' or the elbow may seem flexed (bent).

Arm and hand one-sidedness is usually picked up before the child starts to stand or walk. If it is not, however, you may find that he or she shows different patterns of leg movement between the two sides. By around eight months you may see a baby sitting asymmetrically, tucking one leg up underneath and holding the other out rigidly. However, the motor effect of the hemiplegia on the legs generally becomes obvious when the child starts to move. As we have said, although developmental motor milestones are usually normal or near normal (unless the neurological damage is very severe), the child will often be walking with a limp or tiptoeing, and poor balance, tripping and stumbling are all common.

In congenital hemiplegia it is unusual to find movement of the face affected, except for a mild weakness of the facial muscles or a squint, which is transiently seen in about one in five children that go on to develop hemiplegia. It is even rarer if the hemiplegia originates from early development in the womb. This is very different from acquired hemiplegia, in which it is common to see facial weakness.

The motor signs of weakness, tightness, poor control and increased tendon reflexes (e.g. knee jerks) can be very mild in some children. Dystonia, if there has been involvement of the deep basal ganglia, becomes evident only after about 18 months of age. This is because the basal ganglia motor pathways themselves have not developed until that time so that features of tightness and weakness are initially seen rather than patterns of fluctuating muscle tone.

In some cases of hemiplegia the signs are so subtle that diagnosis can take years. It often comes to light only when the child sees a specialist for another clinical problem, such as epilepsy or a visual difficulty, or when a limb is growing more slowly.

Other clinical problems associated with congenital hemiplegia
As we have seen, it is chiefly the motor areas of the brain that tend to be affected by problems of brain formation or interrupted blood supply. However, all the primary *sensory, communication, cognitive* and *emotional* functions of the brain can also be impaired by the damage that causes the hemiplegia in the first place.

To further complicate matters – children grow. Because of the different rates of growth of underlying bone (controlled by hormones) and overlying muscle and tendons (as a result of physical stretching and relaxation) seen on the affected and unaffected sides, a series of *secondary biomechanical* problems can occur (affecting how muscles, tendons and joints work together). We will now go over some of the ways in which children may present and some of the clinical problems frequently associated with hemiplegia.

Electrical phenomena: epilepsy
An *epileptic seizure* is defined as a short-lived change in behaviour or movement arising from an abnormal electrical discharge from the brain. *Epilepsy* is the label when this happens more than once.

We are all 'allowed' one seizure without being labelled as epileptic. Equally, not all short-lived peculiar motor or behavioural events that lead to altered consciousness (*paroxysmal disorders*) are epileptic in origin but can be have other causes. It is important to put it all into perspective:

- About 7% of the UK population as a whole has had one episode of altered consciousness:
    1. 4.5% of the total were epileptic;
    2. the other 2.5% were generally from febrile convulsions, fainting episodes or breath-holding attacks.
- Between six months of age and four years most single seizures are associated with a fever. Outside these ages it is unlikely to be a simple fever seizure. It is difficult to

tease out the difference between faints and fits and so, if they occur, it is important that you seek the advice of a paediatrician.

If one consults the medical literature on the risk of epilepsy in children with hemiplegia, there is a massive difference in the rates of prevalence quoted. However, if there is a structural lesion in the brain, rates are obviously going to be higher than those seen in the population as a whole. Rates in the initial presentation of an acquired hemiplegia are even greater:

- 40–45% of children with congenital hemiplegia have had at least one seizure.
- 19–28% have 'active' epilepsy requiring treatment. Hemiplegia associated with brain malformations and damage to the brain cortex has a much higher rate of active epilepsy than that associated with damage in the basal ganglia. In the latter group rates are near to those expected in the population as a whole.

The type of seizure that is seen depends on the site of the problem in the brain. Generally episodes of stiffness or twitching (*tonic–clonic seizures*) start on the side of the hemiplegia, but can then spread to involve the whole brain, with loss of consciousness or generalized jerky movements. Strange smells or a visual or sensory aura are also often experienced.

Epilepsy in hemiplegia

- About 70% of epilepsy is focal in origin (starts on the one side).
- 5–40% of seizures then progress to generalized events (spread to involve signs on the other side of the brain – vacancy or twitching).
- About 20% of seizures are associated with the child dropping to the floor (drop attacks).
- About 20% of seizures are triggered by a startle response, in which overwhelming sensory input such as a loud noise or bright light sets off the event.

Most other patterns of epileptic seizures are only slightly more frequently observed in children with hemiplegia in comparison with their peer group as a whole. It is important to repeat that the majority of children with hemiplegia do not even have a single seizure, and even then only a minority will go on to have epilepsy. Of that group three-quarters will be easily managed with medication and many others may be helped by surgery or specific diets (e.g. a ketogenic diet – see Chapter 6). However, the low statistical risk is no consolation to the person with *refractory epilepsy* – one that is resistant to treatment.

Sensory problems
It is difficult to assess sensation fully in children, as their understanding of and cooperation with uncomfortable tests are limited. The sensory cortex of the brain, the area that processes information coming from touch, pain and position sensors in the body, is

situated close to the motor cortex. Structural lesions of the brain in the sensory cortex are therefore relatively common. This can be further affected by any visual impairment.

Sensation is impaired in around half of the children with hemiplegia – usually their sense of position, rather than any other, as it is so closely related to movement. Generally, their sense of pain and temperature sensation are not affected. However, parents will have a much better idea than professionals of any particular problems, and it is obviously important to identify these often overlooked difficulties.

Many families find that the child 'ignores' the hemiplegic arm or leg. This *inattention* generally comes from poor touch sensation, and underlines the complex interaction of the motor and sensory components of the central nervous system. Of course, many children appear to ignore their affected arm even when sensation appears to be normal, simply because it is easier to use the other one.

At the basal ganglia – *locomotor driving system* – level (see Chapter 2) sensory stimulus initiates patterns of movement to seek or shy away from touch. If input goes wrong, output becomes even more disrupted, hence the interaction of sensory abnormality and lack of movement. This may seem complicated – but it does go to show how the different functions of the brain can interact and impact on the patterns of movement.

Some children, on the other hand, may be hypersensitive to touch and cannot bear contact with certain textures.

Another effect can be that the messages between the brain and the bladder and lower bowel are affected, and the young child will take longer to be toilet trained than most children of the same age. Normally all children are out of nappies before the age of three years. Lack of continence in a child over the age of five years (boys seem to develop a little later) requires further investigation.

In children as a whole, after the age of five years, up to one child in 25 may have *faecal incontinence*, usually associated with constipation, and up to two in 25 may have day- or night-time wetting, usually the latter. Difficulties in controlling the bowel and bladder can be up to twice as frequent in children with hemiplegia as in those without. In a large study in the Netherlands *urinary incontinence* was seen in 20% of six-year-olds with a hemiplegia. If there are any concerns about this, parents should seek advice from their paediatrician.

Visual problems
Unfortunately these are relatively frequent and poorly diagnosed. The pathways (visual tracts) carrying messages from the eye to the visual cortex of the brain are close to the ventricles, particularly towards the back. Damage in the *periventricular* areas (see Chapter 2), in particular, can lead to the visual tracts being affected:

● All children with hemiplegia should be referred to an ophthalmologist, and if a problem is detected a 'low vision' teacher assessment should be arranged at an appropriate age.

- At least 25% of children with hemiplegia have a visual field defect. This means that their ability to see things in a particular area of vision can be impaired (*hemianopia*: Greek: 'hemi'= half; 'anopia' = visual defect).

- Around one-quarter to one-half have visuospatial difficulties (i.e. difficulties with the visual perception of objects in space), with specific problems in assessing depth of vision (stereopsy). This has a further impact on their movement disability, as it affects their balance and stability. Diagnosing these subtle signs is extremely complex and, once again, concerns raised by parents about the child's perception of space and place in their environment are important cues to investigate.

- Problems with the coordination of the eye muscles are also more common than in the population as a whole – squints inwards (*convergent*), outwards (*divergent*) or fluctuating (*alternating*).

Hearing problems
These are far less frequent than visual problems in hemiplegia, as the parts of the brain involved are not closely related to the motor areas. When present, they are connected with other factors in the child's clinical history, such as prematurity or early meningitis.

Cognitive (learning) difficulties
When addressing problems in learning it is important to think across a variety of skills, including performance, memory and communication abilities – i.e. IQ (intelligence quotient). A lot of psychological and educational studies have looked at these areas in great detail. In people with hemiplegia, as in the population as a whole, the range of IQ varies greatly from low to well above average.

Most studies, however, do show a comparatively lower full-scale IQ score in children with hemiplegia. The complexity, nature and extent of any cognitive difficulties depend on two major neurological factors:

- firstly, the site and size of the physical damage/impairment in the brain;
- secondly, whether epilepsy is present and controlled. The presence of epilepsy makes it more than three times as likely that the child will have learning difficulties.

If the child does not have epilepsy, then performance IQ (e.g. self-organization and visuospatial skills) is the only cognitive factor that has scored on average lower in children with hemiplegia than in typically developing children in a variety of educational studies. However, if epilepsy *is* present, then there are frequently also problems with verbal skills and memory.

On the whole, language and communication skills (verbal IQ) are not as greatly affected in children with congenital hemiplegia as performance skills. Normally the two sides of the brain have different and specific functions, one side dealing with the receiving and understanding of communication and the other with expression of language. However, if there is early damage to the areas of the brain responsible for speech and language, the brain reorganizes and compensates to preserve these vital skills, a process referred to as *neural plasticity* or *neuroplasticity*. This can, however, be at the expense of other higher-level functions, particularly the visuospatial skills discussed above.

Occasionally, muscle weakness in the mouth and throat can lead to a difficulty in articulation of certain sounds.

As there is less potential for neural plasticity as brain development progresses, left-sided cerebral damage later on in childhood – acquired hemiplegia – will result in difficulties with certain aspects of language. The ability of the right side of the brain to reorganize and compensate is also reduced if a young child has seizures. This means that any child with right-sided hemiplegia and epilepsy is at particular risk of language and educational problems.

Emotional difficulties
The primary and secondary effects of a brain impairment on the psychological well-being of the child and family as a whole should not be underestimated. As a clinician who sees hundreds of young people growing up with hemiplegia, I have no doubt that these emotional difficulties have the greatest impact on all concerned, far more than any physical impairment.

As you know, the brain is a complex organ, and any structural damage has direct implications for thought and feeling. As with learning difficulties, the risk of primary problems is related to the position and spread of the brain damage, and also to whether or not the child has epilepsy. The level of IQ itself is also a significant indicator of risk: the lower the IQ, the higher the likelihood of emotional and behavioural problems.

The reported rates of particular problems vary. In one of the largest studies, the London Hemiplegia Register, carried out by Professor Robert Goodman and his team in the 1990s, the frequencies of psychological disorders in children with hemiplegia were as follows:

- about 25%: anxiety or depression;
- about 24%: conduct disorders – problems with disruptive behaviour and irritability;
- about 10%: severe hyperactivity and inattention;
- about 3%: autistic spectrum disorders – a range of problems with obsessive–compulsive stereotypical behaviour and lack of social or verbal communication skills.

   Anxiety The most frequent problems are specific phobias, both common (e.g. spiders, the dark) and unusual (e.g. specific textures, pyjamas) in origin, or separation anxiety. When at its most severe, the child can show general and almost constant signs of distress, with physical symptoms of pain, insomnia and poor concentration.

Challenging behaviour This covers a whole variety of behaviour, from defiance and negativity, through aggression, to, rarely, more serious antisocial problems such as stealing. It is common for children with hemiplegia to have problems with controlling such behaviour. Early on, children may have very severe temper tantrums, and as they grow out of the 'terrible twos and threes', they may develop more specific irritability and a huge reluctance to do as they are asked. These behaviour patterns stem directly from the damage to the areas of the brain involved with their hemiplegia and are caused by problems in the pathways processing emotional behaviour.

> *Thank you so much. I had been thinking for all of these years that her horrid behaviour was because I was a bad mum.*
>
> *Maggie, East Sussex [in tears]*

Hyperactivity and inattention Many children with hemiplegia have concentration and attention difficulties. For this to be classed as a specific disorder, the problems must be general and not related just to one area. The question is: can they stick at something they have chosen to do or do they remain fidgety, restless and distractible? Computer games and cartoon films do not count, as they are designed to be absorbing and rapidly rewarding, unlike most learning.

Autism Autistic spectrum disorders – including Asperger syndrome, in which verbal communication is less badly affected – are ten times more common in children with hemiplegia than in the population as a whole. Infantile autism in its more severe form is, however, rare, with marked language difficulties being very unusual. Most of the problems observed are with obsessive preoccupation with specific interests, such as Thomas the Tank Engine or fire engines, and a lack of social understanding and interaction with other children of their age.

Secondary/reactive behavioural problems It can feel rubbish having a disability. At school anything that makes you different from your classmates sets you up for an increased risk of teasing, bullying and difficult peer relationships. Add to this the stresses of the academic environment, and the fact that it can take you a long time to do many simple tasks – and it's tough.

Often children will manage to keep their emotions in check while in school, but the pent-up stress means that those with whom they feel most at ease – parents and siblings – get both barrels of anger and frustration when they come back home. Because of this, there is also a very mildly increased risk of some other issues such as obsessive–compulsive behaviours (playing out the stresses), depression (high levels of anxiety) or sadness and anorexia nervosa (especially in teenage girls).

Secondary physical problems
As children with hemiplegia grow, on top of their primary neurologically based problems, they are likely to develop *secondary* physical difficulties (i.e. resulting from the primary, or fundamental, problems). These are, in part, the outward signs of abnormal muscle and tendon growth, and reduced bony *remodelling* (reshaping, formation of new bony tissue) caused by this abnormal growth.

As I have already explained (page 12), bones generally grow because hormones stimulate the cells in the growth plate at their top and bottom to divide. Secondary remodelling of the bone then occurs as a result of the stresses and strains put upon them by the overlying muscles and tendons, creating strong healthy structures. The growth of the overlying muscles and tendons is not under hormonal control but relies on physical stretching and relaxation to stimulate their growth plate, which is positioned where the muscle and tendon meet.

If muscles are fired up all the time because the message from the brain is left on, they cannot stretch and relax appropriately, and then they grow more slowly than the bones. This leads to a tightness that is no longer stretchable but is fixed in a *contracture*.

With these secondary changes to bone and muscle two things can happen:

- Early on, as the child grows, the affected limbs can grow more slowly. In most children there is a couple of centimetres' difference in *true leg length* (measured from the top of the bony hip bone – *anterior superior iliac spine* – to the inside bony bump of the ankle) and perhaps one or two shoe sizes before the age of eight years. It is rare that the difference increases much after that age. The shortening in the arm, hand and fingers can, however, be more pronounced.
- Individual muscles and tendons can restrict the amount of movement across joints, a tight contracture can form in them, and the capsule and ligaments of the joint can further restrict movement. However, the risk of the child developing a secondary curvature of the spine is only slightly higher than in the population as a whole.

Acquired hemiplegia – how it may present
The signs and symptoms of acquired hemiplegia depend on the cause. Often that is a medical emergency, and the specific hemiplegia comes to light only once the initial symptoms have been dealt with.

You may want to flick quickly back to Chapter 3 (pages 22–25) to remind yourself of the causes of acquired hemiplegia so that this section makes sense. Symptoms may include the following:

- A high temperature, seizures or a coma, indicating the presence of an infection of the brain or meninges (the membranes surrounding the brain).
- Post-infective autoimmune disorders may appear after the initial infection, such as measles or chicken pox, has disappeared.
- Worrying signs of severe sudden vomiting, headaches, blurred vision, seizures or coma may indicate raised pressure within the skull. One possible cause of this is a tumour. Once these emergency signs of raised intracranial pressure have been dealt with, signs of a hemiplegia may come to light.
- Vascular, haemorrhagic and clotting problems may already be expected in children with complex cardiac difficulties or a diagnosed bleeding disorder. The sudden

appearance of a dense, specific neurological problem generally means that there has been an acute blockage of one of the main blood vessels to the brain – normally the middle cerebral artery. Seizures can accompany this sudden weakness, and the initially floppy involved limb is slow to develop signs of stiffness. Unlike in congenital hemiplegia, facial weakness is the rule rather than the exception.

- An intermittent fluctuating neurological weakness can be the presentation of some of the incredibly rare progressive forms of acquired hemiplegia, such as loss of cells in *demyelinating disease* (in which the myelin sheath of the nerve fibres is lost, impairing the conduction of signals in the nerves).
- Hemiplegia associated with epilepsy is seen immediately after the seizure and does not get better spontaneously. Most children will go on to have poorly controlled seizures.
- Obvious trauma.

Most acquired hemiplegia occurs before three years of age. The development of signs is rapid: weakness is at its maximum from the beginning, and includes facial weakness. The degree of motor disorder tends to be higher than in congenital hemiplegia, owing to the lack of neural plasticity in the more developed brain.

Other clinical problems associated with acquired hemiplegia

That lack of neuroplasticity in the brain beyond 18 months to three years of age means that the rates and extent of most clinical problems tend to be greater than in congenital hemiplegia. Seizures occur slightly more often, but rates do depend on the underlying cause. Once the initial medical emergency has been resolved, sensory loss, learning difficulties and emotional problems are also seen slightly more frequently.

As stated above, but it is relevant and so bears repeating, if an acquired hemiplegia results from left-hemisphere damage there tends to be a loss of language skills. Unfortunately, the child may also lose previously acquired skills.

Most of the resources listed at the end of chapters are relevant to both congential and acquired hemiplegia. However, the organisations below offer specialised services for people with an acquired brain injury (ABI) such as acquired hemiplegia.

Child Brain Injury Trust (www.childbraininjurytrust.org.uk; helpline 0845 601 4939; email helpline@cbituk.org) provides support to families all over the UK where there is a child with ABI. Services include activity events, legal support, a small grants programme and an 'In Touch' project to put families in touch with one another.

The Children's Trust (www.the childrenstrust.org.uk) offers both residential and community rehabilitation services for children and young people with ABI.

Headway (www.headway.org.uk; Helpline 0808 800 2244; email helpline@headway.org.uk is the main UK support organisation forABI. It is aimed mainly at adults but has useful general information.

Summary
- Hemiplegia is so much more than just a motor disorder.
- The signs of a congenital hemiplegia may not be obvious before one year of age, because the motor system is not sufficiently mature for signs to develop.
- A specific history of prematurity or birth trauma, which may prompt brain scans, can give a clue before signs develop.
- In congenital hemiplegia, signs come to light with asymmetrical, rather than slow, motor development:
  - one-sided handedness before one year of age;
  - asymmetric sitting, standing and walking.
- Other clinical and developmental problems can be seen more frequently in children with hemiplegia than in typically developing children:
  - Epilepsy;
  - sensory difficulties, including visual field and visuospatial problems;
  - specific learning difficulties;
  - emotional and psychological problems, especially anxiety and irritability and obstructive behaviour.
- An acquired hemiplegia generally presents either with the onset of serious whole-body signs or with unilateral weakness, often involving the face. Children are usually very ill.

Chapter 5
After diagnosis – what next?*

Liz Barnes

Don't panic! You are not alone. There is help out there.

Everyone is entitled to grieve over their child's diagnosis, but the best gift you can give yourselves and your child is to accept the disability and love your child for who they are.

At first you don't know what to do, and it's devastating. You are waiting to feel 'normal' again – actually what will happen is that you will develop a 'new normal'.

Finding out that your child has hemiplegia is indeed devastating, although if you have been anxious about him or her 'in the dark' it may also come as a relief to have a name to attach to the worrying signs. In any case, when you have been given the diagnosis you will probably be in a state of shock and confusion. It will be some time before you can think through what this will mean to you and your family. But there is help available, whether it be a question of treatment for your child, problems with money, or just the need to chat to someone who has been through the same experience. Treatment will be offered immediately; other things may have to be asked, or even fought, for, but there are people around to give help and support through this difficult time.

Treatment
When a child is diagnosed with hemiplegia, he or she will normally be referred to the nearest child development centre (CDC) or the child development unit (CDU) at the local hospital. You may indeed receive your diagnosis there. Your general practitioner will of course continue to deal with your child's normal ailments, immunisations, and

---

* By the time you read this, some of the details of benefits and so on may have changed. To find out more go to the Handbook Update page at www.hemihelp.org.uk.

so on, but more specific care will be in the hands of the team at the CDC/CDU, who will refer onwards to other hospital specialists when necessary.

The team at the CDC/CDU will usually include a paediatrician (a specialist in children's medicine who will oversee the child's progress and development), a physiotherapist, an occupational therapist (OT), a speech and language therapist, a psychologist, an orthotist and a social worker. What each of these people does is explained in Chapter 6. During the early years they will play an important role in the life of the whole family, not just treating the child but supporting the parents and teaching them what they can do at home to help develop their son's or daughter's abilities.

CDC/CDUs are friendly, informal places where staff are happy to answer questions and help parents with the anxiety that they are bound to be feeling. You should never be afraid to ask questions, and ask again if you do not understand the answer. Many CDC/CDUs also run groups where parents can meet and support one another.

> *Talk to professionals as much as possible. Get as much information as possible. Join HemiHelp and meet other parents/children as much as possible so you don't feel alone.*

> *There are many parents going through the same situation as you: find a support group.*

At this time you will be giving a lot of time and energy to exercising at home with your child, although much of what you do can be incorporated into play and other everyday activities, and the whole family can be roped in to help. At the same time, you need to be patient, take things one step at a time and enjoy the progress your child is making, however slow. Don't expect doctors and therapists to be able to tell how a child will progress, as each child's hemiplegia is different. Hemiplegia is what is called a *chronic* condition: it will not get better, but your child can be helped to get the best use of the affected arm and leg, and will find all sorts of ways of getting around the practical challenges that life throws at them. Believe it or not, you can tie shoelaces with one hand!

> *Take things one day at a time and celebrate what your child can do, not what they can't do.*

Hemiplegia also does not get worse, but its effects may become more obvious as time goes on. Your child may have difficulties learning to speak, and need speech and language therapy. He or she might be very anxious and clingy, or aggressive and irritable; this is where a psychologist can help. As children with hemiplegia grow, their muscles may become stiffer and they may need more treatment or even surgery, or they may develop epilepsy. Or when they go to school, it may become clear that they have 'invisible' difficulties that get in the way of their learning.

Depending on where the family lives, the CDC/CDU team may care for the child until adulthood, or only until he or she goes to school, when a community team will take over. In that case, therapists may visit the family home or may treat the child at school, especially if he or she has a Statement of Special Educational Needs (see Chapter 8 for more about this).

This all sounds like a good service. Unfortunately, it is not always as good as it should be. Resources vary around the country and, although babies and young children at least should receive very regular therapy (weekly if possible), there is a shortage of qualified therapists and that does not always happen. Almost half of the HemiHelp parent members who filled in our survey form were not satisfied with the frequency of the therapy their child received, especially after reaching school age.

> Up till O attended school we had excellent care and physiotherapy but once at school that really dwindled down.

> Now that J is six, his [occupational therapy] seems to have diminished to three-monthly visits even though he has no use of his left hand and very limited use of his left arm.

A number of parents reported that they had successfully fought for more help, but others have ended up paying for extra therapy or travelling a considerable distance.

In the early years, it is important to keep working at making your baby or toddler use both sides as much as possible, and you can do a lot through play and other daily tasks such as washing, eating, dressing, and so on. HemiHelp also has a DVD, *My Moves*, with useful suggestions for exercising with your child. And, as children grow, formal therapy can often be replaced by sport or other activities that help develop better use of their weaker side and boost their confidence at the same time, as well as being much more fun (see Chapter 7, for more about this).

If you have an appointment to discuss your child's hemiplegia...

- Before your appointment, think about questions you might want to ask and write them down.
- Take someone with you – they will not only give you moral support but can write down what the doctor says.
- If there is anything you want to know or don't understand, just ask, and if you are not happy with the answer ask again until you are.
- Realize that you are the expert on your child and don't be fobbed off – trust your instincts

Other sources of help in the early years

Children's centres
In the past, parents and carers have often been left to find their way, with little help, through a maze of different sources of support (so-called service providers) – social care, health care and so on. However, the UK government has been working to develop a better organized system of help and support for families, including those bringing up a disabled child. In 1999 it launched its first *Sure Start* programmes, which brought together child care, early years education, health care and family support services for families with children under five years. The scheme was first confined to England, and targeted at areas with a high level of child poverty, but its success led to its being extended to cover many more areas.

Now early years programmes are being brought together under one roof in all parts of the UK. The names may be different – children's centres in England and Northern Ireland, integrated children's centres in Wales, family centres in Scotland – and structures and sources of funding vary around the UK and indeed between centres, but the services they provide are similar and may include

- free or affordable play and early education facilities;
- information, support and assistance for parents and carers – including advice on parenting, help with applying for benefits, information on local child-care options and access to specialist services – this may replace the services offered until now by carers' centres, run by some local authorities and charities, notably the Princess Royal Trust for Carers (www.carers.org);
- child and family health services, staffed by health visitors and other professionals, with provision ranging from health and developmental screening to pregnancy and breastfeeding support;
- help for parents wanting to return to work – with links to the local Jobcentre Plus and training;
- toy libraries (www.natll.org.uk), which provide an opportunity to borrow and try out a range of toys that might be useful; specialist play advisors are sometimes available.

Portage (www.portage.org.uk), named after the town in the USA where it started, is a home-visiting educational service with branches all over the UK, where families with a child who has additional needs are visited weekly by trained home visitors who help parents to develop their child's abilities and their own confidence in dealing with everyday challenges.

In England and Wales, the government's **Early Support Programme,** which comes under the Department for Education, is another integral part of services for families with young children with disabilities or emerging special educational needs. Key elements of the programme are

- multi-agency working;
- partnership between service providers and families, with parents at the centre of the planning process;
- the use of key workers to coordinate services for the child; and
- training courses for both parents/carers and professionals

The website (www.education.gov.uk/childrenandyoungpeople/sen/earlysupport; in Wales, www.childreninwales.org.uk/areasofwork/disability/earlysupport/index. html) has an extensive range of resources, with excellent downloadable booklets, including

- an *Early Support: Family Pack* with a background introduction to available services, available in a range of minority languages as well as English, and individual booklets on the social and health services, childcare, financial help, education, etc.;
- information about various types of impairment and living with them, including *Neurological Disorders, Cerebral Palsy, Learning Disabilities, Visual Impairment* and *Autistic Spectrum Disorders*, as well as specific issues e.g. *Sleep, Behaviour;* and
- a set of four developmental journals to help families track, record and celebrate their child's progress through the early years.

Financial and other benefits

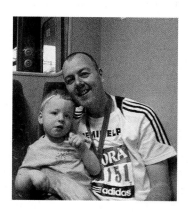

Having a child with a disability can be expensive. Eighty-four per cent of mothers of children with a disability do not work outside the home compared with 39% of mothers of typically developing children. Other mothers and fathers switch from full- to part-time work to give their children the care and attention they feel they need. At the same time, living costs rise: extra heating, extra nappies, adaptations to the home, fuel or public transport fares for hospital visits, and so on. A government survey found that, in 2000, about half of all families with a child with a disability were living in poverty or near to it.

There is financial help available, but you will need to apply for it, and may be turned down or awarded less than you think your child's needs deserve. You may also find that other people have been awarded a higher-rate benefit when their children seem to have the same level of need as your child. But it is possible to appeal, and persistence sometimes pays.

Disability Living Allowance

Disability Living Allowance (DLA) is the main benefit for disabled children. It is usually paid every four weeks and is not means tested – it does not depend on family income or savings. It also does not matter whether parents think of their child as having a disability. For the purposes of DLA, 'disability' simply means that the child has a long-term condition that affects his or her everyday activities.

To get DLA, parents need to fill in a long and detailed application form, which many find very daunting.* But you can get help with this, for example from a health visitor, or someone at the CDC/CDU or a local children's or carers' centre or the Citizens Advice Bureau. Some charities also offer support with applications (see the end of this chapter).

> *Put forward the worst case scenario, i.e. describe your child on a bad day, in order to emphasize the need. Another suggestion would be to diarize what, as parents you do for your child in a day – this will not only emphasize the need but highlight to you, as a parent, what a vital role you play.*

Some children are immediately awarded DLA until they reach the age of 16, but in most cases it is given for two or three years, and then parents need to reapply if they feel that their child still needs extra help. It is worthwhile persisting, and, if necessary, appealing, because receiving any rate of DLA can bring other benefits with it.

DLA has two parts, the care component and the mobility component, and either or both can be claimed:

Care component If the child needs a lot of looking after, or help with personal care, he or she should qualify for the care component. This is payable at three rates, depending on how much extra care the child needs compared with other children of the same age. It can be paid from the age of three months, and it also gives families access to other financial help:

- Getting DLA can lead to extra amounts on other benefits such as Income Support, income-based Job Seekers' Allowance and Housing or Council Tax Benefit.
- It can also lead to increased payments of Working Tax Credit and Child Tax Credit.
- A parent on Income Support or a low wage who spends 35 hours or more a week caring for a child receiving the middle- or high-rate care component may be able to get a Carer's Allowance. This is not a large sum, and may affect other benefits, but the carer is also credited with National Insurance contributions.
- If a child has complex needs, parents may also be entitled to direct payments. These could be appropriate where they are replacing social services support that their child has been assessed as needing, or where they themselves need extra support in their caring role, for example to pay for domestic help or driving lessons. See www.direct.gov.uk/en/CaringForSomeone/CaringForADisabledChild/DG_10018531.
- Parents have slightly improved rights at work regarding parental leave and the right to request flexible working.

Mobility component If the child needs help getting around, he or she may qualify for the mobility component of DLA. The lower rate of mobility component is for children

---

* There are government plans to replace this process with a formal medical assessment from 2013. Go to the Handbook Update page at www.hemihelp.org.uk

who can walk but who may need someone to supervise or guide them. The earliest that this can be paid is from the age of five years. The higher rate is for those who may be unable to walk or have severe difficulties in walking. The earliest this can be paid is from the age of three years. Getting the higher rate for mobility also means that

- parents can apply to their local authority (in Northern Ireland to the Northern Ireland Roads Service) for a Blue Badge for free disabled parking, an on-street parking bay and road tax exemption. You can in fact apply for a Blue Badge as soon as your child is two years old, or earlier if he or she needs bulky 'medical equipment' that cannot be carried around easily – a special car seat, for example;
- a parent can apply to the Department for Work and Pensions to become their child's appointee – a person legally appointed to act on the child's behalf – and hire or hire purchase a car through Motability (www.motability.co.uk), an independent charity set up as a partnership between the government and the charitable and private sectors to help people with disabilities become mobile;
- young people receiving the high rate of the mobility component can become the envy of their friends by taking their driving test at 16, although if they have epilepsy they need to have been free of seizures for a year.

You may still qualify for a Blue Badge without high-rate DLA – contact your local authority for details.

Other financial help

The Family Fund (www.familyfund.org.uk), a government-supported charity, can make grants to families on a low income with children with a disability (aged under 18) to help with the cost of such things as washing machines, computers and other equipment, driving lessons for parents/carers, hospital visiting costs and holidays.

Cerebra (www.cerebra.org.uk), a charity for brain-injured children and young people, can provide grants for equipment and therapies.

Disabled Facilities Grants (in Scotland, **Home Improvement Grants**) are available for families who need to make alterations to their home. If it is a child (under 19) who has the disability, the grants are not means tested. Contact your local authority.

Travelling to hospital There is help with fares to and from hospital for families on income support and low wages. Enquire at the hospital.

Railcard Five- to 16-year-olds may qualify for a disabled person's railcard. They then pay the normal child's fare, but an adult travelling with them gets one-third off the standard adult fare.

Bus travel Reduced fares may also be available for disabled children on local bus services. Contact your local authority.

VAT relief Certain types of equipment (including cars) are free from VAT (value added tax) if they are bought for the use of someone with a disability. This can also apply to building work to adapt your home. You can find more details at www.hmrc.gov.uk/vat/sectors/consumers/disabled.htm.

The following concessions may also be available:

- Some local authorities offer concessions on entry to leisure centres and swimming pools to a child with a disability and a carer.
- Discounts are often available for people with disabilities and their carer(s) on 'days out'. Big attractions such as Chessington World of Adventure, Thorpe Park, and so on, offer wristbands giving priority access to rides – so there is no need to queue. The wristbands are for the person with the disability and up to three or four carers, depending on the ride. Check the park website before you go.
- Theatres, concert halls, museums, etc., usually give a discount, or a free ticket for a carer.
- Most national cinema chains are members of a scheme whereby, if a person with a disability buys a ticket, a carer goes free. Forms can be downloaded from www.ceacard.co.uk to apply for a plastic card. This is not free but will pay for itself after one visit.

For all these concessions, proof of disability is normally required, for example a Blue Badge or evidence that the child or young person receives DLA. Some local authorities have schemes whereby children with disabilities (whether or not they receive DLA) have a card entitling them to concessions.

The legal framework – rights and equality

All the help and services that families and children receive, whether to do with health, education, benefits or just plain everyday life, work within the framework of the law. And here things have definitely been changing for the better.

Traditionally, people have thought about disability using what is now called the 'medical model'. This basically defined people by what they could not do. Take something as basic as climbing stairs: in the past children with mild hemiplegia, who could manage stairs and persuade their friends to carry bags and help them in practical lessons, were able to go to mainstream schools, take exams and get jobs that reflected their abilities. Those who had difficulty with stairs or balance might find themselves in a special school where their academic abilities might not be developed to the full and their future job prospects limited.

People who had difficulty walking also had problems going to see a play or a film or a football match, because 'what would happen if there was a fire and they couldn't move fast enough?' As for using public transport, they could forget it. Disability was also often seen as shameful or comic, and families were put off taking their child out, knowing that they would be stared or laughed at.

Of course, attitudes take time to change, and parents sometimes still complain about how their children are treated when they go out, but this is no longer seen as normal. Public transport authorities in the UK now have to ensure that new buses and trains are accessible, and schools can no longer turn children away because they cannot climb stairs easily.

Behind these changes is a change in the way we see disability. The medical model is gradually being replaced by the 'social model'. This says that everyone, whatever their abilities or disabilities, has equal rights as a human being and a citizen, and the world around them has to change to allow them to exercise these rights. It might be something simple such as a lift or a ramp, it could be something much more difficult such as changing how people think, or how they talk, but it is happening.

The Equality Act 2010
In the UK, as in many other countries, this change has been reflected in laws designed to end discrimination on the grounds of disability – laws that came about largely thanks to the efforts of the people with disabilities themselves. In the UK the Disability Discrimination Act (DDA) was first passed in 1995 and then amended several times as new areas of life were added to those covered by the Act. In 2010 all these changes became part of the Equality Act, which brought together and strengthened earlier antidiscrimination measures affecting different groups of people into one single law intended to benefit everyone.

The Equality Act covers a range of areas, including

- employment,
- health care,
- education,
- access to goods, facilities and services, and
- buying or renting land or property.

One important area of the law for children with hemiplegia and their families is the one that deals with education. This is because more and more children with disabilities and additional needs now go to mainstream schools, which are having to adapt both their buildings and their attitudes. Many children with hemiplegia manage well at school, with or without support, but some parents feel that their child is not getting the help he or she needs and would like to know more about their rights. See Chapter 8 for more about this.

The Equality Act also includes for the first time the rights of carers as a separate group. In 2008 a British woman had to appeal to the European Court of Justice after resigning from her job because her employer would not allow her to work flexibly in order to look after her disabled son. She won her case, and, thanks to input from disability groups during the drafting of the Equalities Act, people in her situation are now protected from discrimination by UK law.

Adults with hemiplegia may want to know more about their rights under the Equality Act on a range of issues. See Chapter 9 for more on this.

Local and national support groups

In this chapter I have written about various kinds of support given by people working in health and social services and other professionals. But for families in which there is a child with hemiplegia the best support often comes from people like themselves – parents helping parents through a crisis, or children discussing their lives with other children. This may be face to face, by telephone or online, using email, Twitter, Facebook or a forum or message board.

> *Join a local special needs group. It's good to be with others who have similar needs and you can support each other.*

Children with hemiplegia live all around the country, but each one will probably be the only person at their school with the condition, and families may not know of anyone else with hemiplegia in their area. But this does not have to be a problem: people dealing with a disability in their lives have a lot in common, even if it is not the same disability. They will all be trying to get the best out of the health and education systems, looking for sports and other activities for their children, coping with their child's and their own anxieties, and sometimes getting just plain exhausted in the process. You may find a support group for another condition, or a group where there are people living with various different conditions. Many CDC/CDUs run groups where parents can find support from one another, or will know of groups in the area. Your local children's centre may provide support and practical help for carers. See below for other ways to find groups close to you. And if you cannot find a group in your area, you can always start one up!

National organizations

HemiHelp
www.hemihelp.org.uk
0845 120 3713 (office)
0845 123 23720 (helpline)
support@hemihelp.org.uk

HemiHelp is the national organization in the UK for children and adults with childhood-onset hemiplegia and their families. It was founded in 1990 by a handful of London parents who met because their children were taking part in Professor Robert Goodman and Dr Carole Yude's research into the causes and effects of childhood hemiplegia. Finding out how helpful it was to share their anxieties and experience, they decided to set up a group to offer support and information to other parents in the same situation. Like a lot of charities, HemiHelp was run for many years entirely by volunteers, most of them parents, and using the attic of a founder member as headquarters. However, it has now grown into a national organization with professional staff and a membership of around 3600 families, medical and educational professionals, and adults with hemiplegia.

HemiHelp receives no government funding, and is financed from a wide range of sources, including grants from charitable trusts, donations from companies, fundraising concerts and other events. Members themselves are also important here, whether organizing coffee mornings or taking part in sponsored sporting events such as the London Marathon. These efforts are valuable not only for the income they produce but also because they raise awareness of hemiplegia.

HemiHelp has close links with other disability organizations in the UK and other countries and with specialists in various aspects of the condition. But becoming larger and more professional does not mean that it has lost contact with its roots. A majority of its trustees are still parents of children with hemiplegia or adults with the condition, and members are very much at the heart of all its services and activities.

HEMIHELP SERVICES
- A telephone/email information and support service staffed by volunteers who are either parents or adults with hemiplegia.
- A home visitor service to help solve more complex problems.
- Training to help schools support pupils with hemiplegia.
- An extensive website with a members' message board.
- A Facebook group and a Twitter feed (@hemihelp).
- Putting members in touch with others who have faced similar difficulties and developing a network of local groups.
- A regular magazine in which members can read about new developments in research and treatments, get practical information and advice on living with hemiplegia, and share their own concerns and experiences.
- Information sheets and booklets on subjects of interest to members, downloadable for free from the website.
- An online shop selling the *Primary Schools Pack* and other publications, as well as the *My Moves* physiotherapy DVD and a range of equipment to help people with hemiplegia in their daily lives.
- Regular conferences and workshops for parents and professionals around the UK and in the Republic of Ireland.
- Sports and activity fun days and music and drama workshops for children in different regions.

Here are some comments from HemiHelp's survey of its members, which show how its services have helped them:

> L met other children with hemiplegia, both at the music workshop and the fun day. This helped her to realize she was not the only one with a funny hand.

> The fun day gave A contact with other kids like himself. Gave us support and insight into the condition.

> Leaflets to hand out to carers, friends and relatives, website for reading other scenarios. Fun days are excellent – to feel normal for the day.

A constant source of information and reassurance that you are not the only one.

It is lovely to read about others with hemiplegia who have led normal lives and have good jobs. It helps us to be positive about H's future.

Phoned helpline in tears, spoke to lovely woman. Made us realize we're not alone.

No one explained the behaviour stuff – luckily HemiHelp did – this probably kept our family together.

It has made me into a fighter for my child, being able now to go anywhere and fight anyone for what I believe are his rights.

Scope
www.scope.org.uk
0808 800 3333 (Scope Response)
response@scope.org.uk

Scope (formerly the Spastics Society) was founded in 1952 and is the main national organization for people with cerebral palsy of all types.

SCOPE SERVICES
● Practical services in areas such as education, employment and independent living, in both disabled and mainstream settings.
● Scope Response, a freephone and email information, advice and support service (see above).
● A live web chat service for families with disabled children, run by trained Relate counsellors.
● A wide range of downloadable information and fact sheets, including some produced in conjunction with HemiHelp.
● Community development teams who support a network of over 250 affiliated local groups and work to develop local services and projects.
● Support for face2face (www.face2facenetwork.org.uk; 0844 800 9189), a one-to-one befriending service for parents of children with disabilities.
● Campaigns for disabled rights and equality.

Contact a Family (CAF)
www.cafamily.org.uk
0808 808 3555 (helpline)
helpline@cafamily.org.uk

Contact a Family offers support, advice and information to families with children with disabilities, no matter what their condition or disability, and also to the professionals who work with them. As well as an excellent website with downloadable booklets and leaflets on a wide range of subjects, it has a network of national, regional, and local project offices that provide local disability information, support parent groups in their area, and run activities such as workshops and family events. It also has a network of volunteer local representatives who are parents of children with disabilities and can help with local contacts and support. Additionally, helpline advisers can arrange an interpreter over the phone for parents who do not speak English.

Cerebra
www.cerebra.org.uk
0800 328 1159 (helpline)
info@cerebra.org.uk

Cerebra is a charity that offers information and support service for parents, carers, and others involved with any child or young person with a brain-related condition. It has a range of fact sheets, including an excellent guide to claiming Disability Living Allowance, runs a postal book library and has a number of regional offices. It can also give grants for certain kinds of equipment and therapy.

Dial UK
www.dialuk.info
01302 310 123 (office)
informationenquiries@dialuk.org.uk

This is a network of 140 local disability information and advice line services run by and for disabled people.

Gingerbread
www.gingerbread.org.uk
0808 802 0925 (helpline)

This organization offers information and advice to lone parents

Mumsnet
www.mumsnet.com

This is a popular social network site for parents with lots of useful general information. Its *Special Needs* page has articles on diagnosis, benefits, education etc. Go to *Mumsnet Talk* to join an online discussion (includes a thread for disabled parents).

Scotland
Capability Scotland
www.capability-scotland.org
0131 337 9876
ascs@capability-scotland.org.uk

Capability Scotland was set up to support people with cerebral palsy, but has developed to support children, young people and adults with a range of disabilities. One of

Scotland's leading disability organizations, it provides a diverse range of services including community living, day and residential services, employment, respite/short breaks, therapy, education and learning, family support, and activities. Its very useful website has downloadable publications and fact sheets on many subjects, including equipment, holidays and leisure activities, and a wide range of links.

Kindred
www.kindred-scotland.org
0131 536 0583 (helpline)
kindred.enquiries@gmail.com

Run mainly by parents and based at an Edinburgh hospital, KINDRED (formally known as SNIP) provides advice and information on services available to children with additional support needs and their carers, and provides a 'listening ear'.

Where to find out about benefits and other types of support

Directgov (www.direct.gov.uk) is the single point of online access to government services and information, including carers' and disability services and information – covering financial support, rights, independent living and much more. Useful sections include www.direct.gov.uk/carers and www.direct.gov.uk/disability.

Benefits enquiry (freephone 0800 882 200; Northern Ireland 0800 220 674): go to www.dwp.gov.uk/eservice/ to fill in or download a DLA form

Citizens Advice Bureau (www.adviceguide.org.uk) for help with benefits, rights, etc. The home page will direct you to pages for all parts of the UK.

Disability Alliance (www.disabilityalliance.org): a charity with the principal aim of improving the living standards of disabled people. Publications include the *Disability Rights Handbook* and a range of useful fact sheets and other information on such things as direct payments, tax credits and the Employment and Support Allowance.

Other useful sites include the following:

Advice Now (www.advicenow.org.uk): follow the link to *Sickness and disability benefits*.
Benefits and Work (www.benefitsandwork.co.uk).
Benefits Now (www.benefitsnow.co.uk).
Turn2Us (www.turn2us.org.uk).

Advice, information and campaigning for carers

Care Coordination Network UK (ccnukorguk.site.securepod.com; info@ccnuk.org.uk): this is a networking organization promoting and supporting care coordination or key working for disabled children and their families. The site has a dad's page with useful links for fathers.

Carers UK (www.carersonline.org.uk).

Carers Scotland (www.carerscotland.org).

Carers Wales (www.carerswales.org).

Carers N Ireland (www.carersni.org).

Summary
- When you find out your child has hemiplegia, you will be devastated and confused, but you should take one day at a time and remember that there is help available.
- After diagnosis, your child will be referred to the multidisciplinary team at your local Child Development Centre (CDC) or hospital Child Development Unit (CDU), who will take charge of treatment for his or her hemiplegia.
- CDC/CDUs are friendly places: don't be afraid to ask questions, and ask again until you understand the answers.
- The therapists at the CDC/CDU will show you how to work with your child at home to help him or her become as two-sided as possible.
- Much of this can be done through play activities and can involve the whole family.
- Your CDC/CDU may also have a parents' group, where you can share your concerns and experiences with people who are going through the same difficult times.
- Your local children's centre will also be a useful source of information and support.
- Having a child with a disability means having extra expenses, but there is financial help available.
- The main form this takes is Disability Living Allowance (DLA), which has two components, for care and mobility, and different levels depending on the severity of your child's disability.
- Receiving DLA at any level may give you access to other benefits.
- Receiving the DLA mobility component at the high rate allows you to lease a car from Motability. You can also have a Blue Badge, which will give you free parking and exemption from road tax.
- You may have to fight to get your child the help you need, but there are many UK charities offering information and support for families where there is a child with a disability.
- HemiHelp and Scope are the specialist organizations for hemiplegia and cerebral palsy, but other charities (for example those that deal with benefits and how to claim them) can also be helpful.
- Above all, remember your child is always your child. He or she may take longer to reach the usual milestones, but each achievement, however small, will bring you joy.

Chapter 6

Assessment and clinical management

Charlie Fairhurst

As parents we tend to go to the internet, but because we don't really know what we're looking at we sometimes look in the wrong direction at stuff that's not appropriate. You end up not having a clue and scaring yourself half to death.

Susan and Adam, Hampshire

In this very long chapter, you may want to dip in and out of sections as they become relevant. You might find us using 'medic speak' such as 'intervention' where you would expect 'treatment' or 'limbs' rather than 'arms' and 'legs'. I have tried to achieve a balance between using the terminology that you will inevitably hear professionals using and the more everyday words that you might use yourself.

As a parent, everyone that you meet at any point of your child's *clinical pathway* is an expert in his or her own field. Do not forget, however, that you are, in turn, the world expert on your own child. The fundamental requirement for the holistic well-being of any child is balanced, thoughtful, open communication between parents and professionals.

Balanced For both, having the appropriate knowledge, what is proven and what is not.

Thoughtful For both, able to listen when appropriate, talk when appropriate, and then reflect to make the best decision for the individual child.

Open For both, mutual respect, thinking about the child first and foremost.

Communication For the professionals, the ability to foster mutual understanding rather than hiding behind terms and phrases. I have been in professional meetings in which everyone believes that they have said the same things, but the parents and, in fact, everyone else end up confused. The doctors might as well have been speaking Russian, the therapists French, Italian and Spanish, the care staff Chinese and the teachers Hindi.

Until the time that a child reaches 'competence' to make his or her own choices, the parent is the advocate, i.e. the decision-maker and provider of consent for any intervention. Knowledge is the key to taking on that role. In health care internationally, we talk now about the *patient pathway*. Basically it means who, what, when and why: the points at which people and clinical interventions may become appropriate to help minimize the impact of a condition on a person's physical and psychological well-being.

That is what we are going to talk about now, the ifs, whats and whens of best assessment and treatment options – evidence-based practice, clinical governance, and other buzz phrases.

Remember, we cannot do anything (yet) about the primary brain impairment, so we are attempting to treat the secondary motor and other clinical problems.

The clinical patient pathway

We are all individuals, and therefore the point at which someone with hemiplegia enters the health system will vary – as we have seen with the possible ways of presentation in Chapter 4. To recap, presentation of congenital hemiplegia may come through an obstetric or baby unit, but generally it comes from concern about *asymmetry* of function (unevenness in the development of the child's left and right side) at some point in infancy.

In the UK there are various points at which health visitors – specialist nurse practitioners in the community – and general practitioners are responsible for screening the development of all children. These occur generally around six weeks and eight and 18 months. A range of developmental skills are looked at to ensure that there is neither an imbalance between the two sides of the child nor any developmental delay compared with the child's wider peer group.

As an asymmetry of motor control, congenital hemiplegia should be picked up by the professionals at one of these standardized screening stages, but subtle differences may become visible only much later. It is, however, much more likely that the parents themselves will be concerned about the pattern of their child's movement and will seek referral from their general practitioner. Trainee paediatricians are always told, 'The parent knows best' – so you should expect to have your thoughts taken very seriously.

Team-working in health services

In any team sport, a successful team is made up of individuals, all of whom are skilled individuals in their position or function but who also bring their own particular strength to the team. The same principle applies in the health service.

There is no point being an individual in a football team, and the same goes for the health service. Any successful team that helps and supports a child through his or her growth and development must be multidisciplinary to the core. Appropriate management of any child with hemiplegia can happen only with such a team approach, keeping the child and family at the centre of any decision-making process.

As a paediatrician I am dependent on the expertise of colleagues in other medical disciplines, such as orthopaedic surgeons and ophthalmologists, as well as many other experts in fields such as gait analysis, physiotherapy occupational, speech and language and psychotherapy, and orthotics – as well as nursing specialists, 'alternative' therapists, teachers and social workers.

Once you have seen the health visitor and your general practitioner, the next point of call in the UK should be the local child development centre (CDC), the core of community health services. If any child has a problem that is primarily developmental, then this is the key route – not to a hospital paediatrician or orthopaedic surgeon first off, a side turning that can often add months to the time taken to get appropriate assessment and intervention.

A 'who's who' of the child development centre

Although we will go through the roles one by one, what is important is that all these individuals work in a multidisciplinary team:

- assessing the child as part of the family;
- making individual tailored management plans with the child and family, prioritizing areas of functional difficulty;
- setting realistic goals with the child and family and the rest of the multidisciplinary team;
- intervening and implementing the management plan; and
- reviewing the management plan on a regular basis, often using specific assessment systems as outlined later.

Manager/administrator

- The glue that holds the team together.
- Coordinates everything to do with the service, from stationery deliveries through to appointments and maternity leave cover.

Nursery nurse/nurse and play specialist

- Provides support for all services, as well as leading various groups and interacting with parents, often as the first point of contact. Helps provide practical knowledge about child development and welfare, based on a wealth of experience built up from a good grounding in theory.
- Has specialist knowledge in other areas of concern such as nutrition, various clinical conditions and the practical aspects of bringing up a child with a developmental disability.
- Provides guidance on using play as a therapeutic approach.

Physiotherapist

- In a child with a movement disorder, assessment, intervention and review by the physiotherapy team is key.
- Undoubtedly the member of the team with the widest knowledge of motor development, ability and function, and therefore best placed to advise on the correct management.
- Focuses particularly on body and leg and foot posture, balance and movement.
- Professional lead on goal setting and planning for motor ability; therefore often the first point of call between the child and the family and the rest of the service.
- Involved in many different practical assessments, and specific approaches to therapy.
- Aims to minimize secondary deformity at the level of muscles and tendons by targeted strengthening and stretching, promoting activity and balance.
- Together with the occupational therapist and orthotist, often advises on, assesses and 'tweaks' specific pieces of equipment, such as casts and splints.
- Focuses on the treatment of reduced sensation, hypersensitivity and visuospatial difficulties, together with the occupational therapist.
- As resources are limited, trains and supports parents in a home programme of therapy (to give the child the best possible function on the affected side).

Occupational therapist

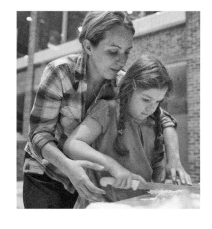

- Focuses on how to improve a child's function through play, learning and home life.
- Educates and supports parents directly in how to minimize the impact of arm and hand difficulties.
- Aims to minimize problems arising from visuospatial perception difficulties in the child's environment and work on ways to enable the child to participate at home and school.

- Assesses the need for and provides special equipment across all areas of home and school life in order to make all activities of daily living as easy as possible, helping the child to gain independent living skills.

Speech and language therapist

- Assesses and manages all aspects of communication. This may include language understanding, the development of speech (articulation) and expressive language (learning words and putting sentences together, and how language is used for learning and social communication). Also considers non-verbal communication such as eye contact, facial expression and gestures.
- Some specialize in the assessment and treatment of eating, drinking and swallowing and saliva control.
- May work in community clinics, nurseries, schools and hospitals: may be involved with all age ranges, from babies with feeding difficulties to adults with specific learning disorders.

Psychologist

- Not all CDCs have one: if there is one, he or she will assess and intervene in any emotional and behavioural problems associated with hemiplegia, providing critical support, understanding, and practical approaches for the children and their families.

Community paediatrician

- Doctor specializing in children – diagnoses, organizes investigations, liaises with specialist and other interdisciplinary services, and coordinates any medical interventions.
- Also responsible for local care pathways and the implementation of health policies.

Other specialists

Many others come to the CDC from time to time, such as orthotists (specialists in the provision of splints), ophthalmologists to check vision, and audiologists to check hearing.

Others may also be called in from other regional services from time to time for specific investigations, advice and interventions. These may include paediatric neurodisability specialists; paediatric neurologists; a movement therapy team, including a gait analysis laboratory team; and orthopaedic surgeons.

Assessments

The team will initially want to find out all about the pregnancy and delivery and look for any risk factors for the various causes of congenital hemiplegia. They will then want to work out the physical signs of the movement disorder, what 'type' of muscle tone is most evident and any other apparent impairment of vision or sensation. Here, we will consider the assessment procedure first and then look at some specific areas.

General movement assessments (including gait analysis)

General movement assessments

- examine active and passive movements;
- examine muscle 'tone' and power;
- look at how the child moves and walks (if appropriate);
- include a functional look at age-appropriate levels of activity/ability.

When the team looks at children's motor ability they need to see them sit, stand and move. The key to all paediatric practice is observation: they will look at how a child is moving and examine the muscle bulk and length of the arms and legs. Mobility can be about more than walking, so it may be appropriate for the team to watch the child crawling, bottom-shuffling or moving in any other way.

However, in walking, there are basically three sections to a step (the *gait cycle*) – strike, stance, and swing. We look at what happens at the body (trunk) level, hips and pelvis, knees, ankles and feet, as well as what the child is doing with his or her arms. It is normal to be symmetrical, so any difference between the two sides is important:

> **Strike** Which part of the foot hits the floor first?
>
> **Stance** What happens at the different levels as the weight is transferred forward, i.e. when the foot is on the ground?
>
> **Swing** How is the foot brought through in order to put it down again?

The team may simply make notes on what they see as they observe the child walking, they may video the child walking, or they may use formal three-dimensional gait analysis. This uses technology similar to that used for animations in films like *Avatar*, *Lord of the Rings*, or *The Lion, the Witch and the Wardrobe*.

Little silver golf ball markers are placed around the child's joints and a room full of infrared cameras pick up their position as he or she walks, to create a computerized model of movement. From this, along with information from a sensitive force plate on the floor, the team can see how all the muscles involved in walking work. When there is a problem, they can work out how much the problem is due to muscle tightness and how much to weakness. That is really important when they are working out how best to try to improve the child's walking.

Part and parcel of any motor assessment is a general physical examination, looking at the child's weight and height and how straight the spine is. In hemiplegia it is important to look at true leg length on both sides (from the top of the bony hip bone to the inside bony lump of the ankle).

Doctors will also examine specific neurological signs, particularly tendon reflexes, muscle tone/stretchability, motor control, including selective movements (active wiggling of feet, toes, knees and hips), active and passive ranges of movement, standing balance, and levels of muscle power. As we have seen in earlier chapters, the muscles tend to be tight and weak and lack coordination on the affected side.

Initially tightness tends to be stretchable or *dynamic*, but over time there is normally a loss in the range of movement, known as *contracture*. The team will look at the joint ranges and record how much tightness and weakness there is in the muscles of the arm and leg.

Mobility and balance can be further affected by visuospatial and sensory difficulties. If these become evident, a review by specialists will be necessary.

Specific movement assessment tests
Many specific assessment tools can then be used by the individual members of the team, focusing on upper and lower limb ability, depending on the age and stage of development of the child. These look at

- active ranges of movement,
- ease and fluidity of motor control,
- dexterity and balance,
- specific task activities, participation and performance,
- function and dysfunction, and
- ability and disability.

These tools can be useful at initial assessment but are particularly relevant when reviewing the benefit of any specific treatment. The following are some of the most common you may come across.

LOWER LIMB ASSESSMENT TESTS
    Gross Motor Function Measure (GMFM) A detailed look at how children aged five to 16 lie, sit, crawl, stand and walk, run and jump in comparison with typically developing children of their own age.

    Timed Up and Go Test (TUG) A simple test of the ability to stand up, walk a small distance, turn round, come back and sit down again.

    Six-minute Walk Test A measure of how far, fast and easily a child can walk.

    Gillette Functional Assessment Questionnaire A very simple way of scoring walking ability, looking at how the child manages with distance, slopes, stairs, uneven surfaces and pavements.

UPPER LIMB ASSESSMENT TESTS

Assisting Hand Assessment (AHA) The child is given toys that encourage two-handed play skills. A video of the session looks at how objects are stabilized, grasped, released, and fiddled with.

Shriner's Hospital Upper Extremity Examination (SHUEE) This does a very similar thing in slightly older children: shoulder, elbow, wrist, finger and thumb movements are studied during tasks requiring both hands.

Melbourne Assessment of Unilateral Upper Limb Function A formal scoring of upper-limb movement in children aged between 2 years 6 months and 15 years.

Other developmental assessments
As we have seen, hemiplegia is far more than a movement disorder, and assessment of vision, sensation, language and emotional difficulties will also be made when relevant. Testing vision is particularly challenging in young children and, if there is any concern, specialist advice from an ophthalmologist would be sought.

Psychologists and other members of the community teams may use a series of specific assessments to pick up emotional and behavioural difficulties, evaluate their extent, and work out a treatment programme.

Investigations
Once the initial developmental and physical check-up has taken place, it may be appropriate for doctors to do some investigations discussed here, to work out why the hemiplegia happened. Other investigations may take place to help with the management of specific complications such as epilepsy.

Neuroimaging: to scan or not to scan?
The advent of detailed neuroimaging (brain scans) dramatically changed how we think about hemiplegia. Nowadays a magnetic resonance image (MRI) of the brain would normally be carried out on all children suspected or confirmed as having hemiplegia.

An MRI scanner uses a large external magnet to detect differences in the electrical charge held by the atoms making up the different fluids and solids within the body, particularly in fat and water. Basically, the moving magnets pick up different cell fluid properties within the brain and thereby create a picture of its anatomy by distinguishing the watery cells from the fatty tracts.

WHY SCAN?
Looking at the extent of the damage in the brain can provide useful information for everyone involved in looking after a child with hemiplegia. It gives us clues to what may have caused the problem and about what the prognosis (future abilities and disabilities) is likely to be. As we saw in Chapter 3, specific brain problems occur at different stages of brain development in the womb, at the time of birth or soon afterwards:

- Early in the womb: brain malformations.

- Very premature: periventricular haemorrhagic infarctions – bleeding into the brain tissue around the ventricles in the centre of the cortex.

- Premature: periventricular leuckomalacia – areas of cell damage leading to loss of cells around the ventricles of the cortex.

- Full term: deep damage to the areas under the brain cortex – the basal ganglia.

- Blood vessel strokes: distinct 'punched out' areas of damage related to the parts of the brain provided by the artery that is blocked or bled.

- Sometimes the scan reveals problems that may have a genetic basis and may therefore have important implications for the child or family.

WHY NOT SCAN?
Most young children need a general anaesthetic for brain MRI. Although the risks associated with an anaesthetic may be small, they are still present. Equally, although the scan may be interesting, it is often only of limited use when deciding how to help the child. (This is not, however, the case if epilepsy is present, when a scan can help with decisions about what medicine is relevant and whether a surgical approach should be considered.)

. . . THAT IS THE QUESTION
Communicate, deliberate, advocate. . .

Blood tests
If there is no clear reason for the hemiplegia, it may be appropriate to do some blood tests. That will be of particular importance if the cause is thought to have been a blockage or haemorrhage from one of the cerebral arteries. In such cases we need to check for a problem with the clotting system of the blood, or other factors that could lead to increased stickiness of the blood. This is particularly important for acquired hemiplegia.

Electroencephalogram (EEG)
If the child is having seizures, the most important factor for diagnosis is a good clinical history. An EEG can be helpful to look at the electrical activity underlying any problem. Surface electrodes are placed on the scalp to record brain activity. However, the recording is only as good as the operator who performs it and the team that interpret it. It is very much like trying to work out what happens in a film by looking at the poster. One can see the main characters and a bit of background but it does not tell one anything about the story – it is simply a snapshot.

Sometimes the scan is normal; sometimes it shows an abnormal electrical trace even when there have been no obvious clinical seizures. Indeed, in hemiplegia this is more than likely to be the case, as with an underlying structural difference there is likely to be an abnormal electrical signal. It can be confusing, and that is why the history is so important. Universal treatment is unnecessary: if we treated all the children with abnormal EEG traces, anticonvulsants would be given to the majority of children with hemiplegia.

Interventions (treatments)

If the history, examination, assessments and investigations have picked up functional problems, the child health team will need to consider how they can focus interventions to minimize any potential disability. In medicine we have to consider what is in the best interests of the patient – evidence-based practice and clinical governance are the current buzz phrases used to describe how this is done.

- Evidence-based medicine simply means basing clinical decision-making on the evidence available from scientifically conducted trials.
- Clinical governance refers to the systematic approach now taken to monitor the quality of patient care in the health service.

Therapy and other treatments change both with the needs of the child and over time. Part and parcel of any intervention is to agree targeted goals with the parents and child. These can then be reviewed after the course of therapy, injections, surgery, or whatever, perhaps by repeating the specific assessments and reappraising the treatment programme. Again, this cycle of appraisal, goal setting, intervention, and reappraisal is key to the clinical patient pathway.

Motor interventions

The principles of motor management focus on the way the hemiplegia affects the individual child. The CDC team has to respond to the dynamic processes of bone, muscle and tendon growth in order to minimize the development of secondary biomechanical deformities. They have to take an adaptive approach, i.e. use the different options available in order to work with, rather than against, the background development of the child's movement and posture.

The core of the patient pathway for any child is coordinated therapy, trying to optimize his or her potential and minimize his or her disability. There are many different approaches to physical and occupational therapy. Individual CDCs will use slightly different methods, but most are based on the principles we have discussed earlier (see page 56): sensory integration in movement, neuroplasticity, patterning, muscle strengthening and stretching. Parents and other carers are taught many of the techniques so that they can continue therapy on a daily basis to maximize ability and minimize disability.

PHYSIOTHERAPY – TO STRETCH OR TO STRENGTHEN?
One thing you learn if you have been part of 'the system' long enough is that what comes around goes around. Twenty years ago, strengthening was the focus of therapeutic options. Ten years ago, stretching was all important. Realistically, a balanced approach of strengthening, stretching, selectivity, and motor fluidity, focusing on goal-orientated activity, is considered far more effective.

● Exercise programmes target specific muscle groups.
● Stretching can be helped by pulses (several short spells) of serial plaster casting across joints or splinting.

Custom-made casts and splints (*orthoses*) hold one part of the body in a particular position. Usually the name describes the part of the body that is being worked on: for example, ankle–foot orthoses (AFO) are splints for the calf and ankle. They apply a constant force in order to stretch muscles. Casts are short-term interventions and splints or orthoses are generally longer term. Some people believe that the child should live in the splints; others feel that their usefulness is limited. My personal opinion is that time in splint helps to stretch, but too much time in them can weaken the muscle further as they tend to prevent active movement. Also, it is worthwhile mentioning that shoe lifts and raises have no proven benefit. Long-term trials show that they do not prevent any spinal curve or prevent any future problems such as osteoarthritis and, if anything, it is felt they increase the level of disability rather than help.

There can be a confusing variability in advice given to parents to do with many movement therapies, particularly the use of splints. Also lack of liaison between various parts of the medical system may sometimes lead to long delays in provision of equipment, so that an orthosis may be outgrown before it arrives.

Strengthening tends to receive less attention than stretching, but, as we have seen, it is just as important. Strength, balance and activity therapy – following other medical treatments, such as botulinum toxin A injections or surgical interventions – are equally important in getting the best result. In this case, one plus one equals three.

Many therapists use specific approaches to therapy. One of the most common is neurodevelopmental therapy – the *Bobath approach* –whereby the therapist tries to modify muscle tone and repeat typical patterns of movement so that the brain learns these patterns and the child begins to use these movements automatically. A similar adaptive approach is used in other widely used techniques, such as *Vojta therapy* or *conductive education*, as championed by the Peto Institute in Budapest. Plasticity within the nervous system is encouraged in all such therapeutic approaches by patterning of movements. The principles have broad acceptance and although there has been an increasing number of studies of these therapies the evidence base to support their benefit, like many interventions for cerebral palsy is not robust.

OCCUPATIONAL THERAPY
Again the cycle of assessment, planning, intervening and re-evaluating is vital. Occupational therapy works on the same principles as physiotherapy, but generally focuses on tasks requiring two hands, encouraging the affected arm to be brought into functional use. Stretching uses splints from a variety of materials, from rigid polypropylene to wetsuit material (neoprene) and Lycra.

The focus of many different treatment approaches is either to use the affected side rather than the 'good' hand – *constraint-induced therapy* – or to bring the affected side into functional two-handed tasks. There are a whole host of ways that one can encourage this through play, education, and targeted programmes such as *HABIT – Hand–Arm Bimanual Intensive Training*. Both of these approaches require a considerable amount of practice every day and can be difficult for young children to tolerate.

Often it is better to persuade the child that therapy is actually play. Different play approaches using repetitive tasks to improve reach and wrist, finger and thumb ability are constantly being re-evaluated. Two that we use increasingly at the Evelina Children's Hospital in London are *magic therapy* and *virtual reality training*. The first encourages children to use both hands to do magic tricks and the second uses the affected arm in combination with virtual reality toys to manipulate play environments. In a home environment the use of specific game consoles such as the Nintendo Wii can be extremely useful in applying therapy through fun activity, using a variety of bilateral hand and arm movements to interact with the screen.

Occupational therapists and physiotherapists vitally support other members of the team, such as parents, care staff, teachers and support assistants, by evaluating what equipment is necessary to help learning and independence at school and home. Therapy teams are also vital in trying to minimize the impact of sensory difficulties and visual problems on activity. Helping a child overcome hypersensitivity in a limb requires great skill and care, as does encouraging him or her to move in an environment when his or her vision is limited.

MEDICAL MOVEMENT THERAPIES (FIGURE 6.1)
As part of the patient pathway doctors can offer several options for 'medical movement therapy', treating the child as a whole (global) or one part (focal), i.e. arm or leg, in a more or less reversible or permanent fashion.

In hemiplegia, focal treatment tends to be a more sensible approach than treating the whole child. I would also stress that any medical treatment works only in combination with, rather than taking the place of, day-to-day therapy.

General medical interventions
I am now going to describe some of the medicines currently used to modify muscle tone and control. But remember -

● they all have significant side effects;
● they work on both sides of the body, and so their use is not always appropriate in hemiplegia. However, occasionally the motor problem on the affected side can be so intense that, on balance, they are needed.

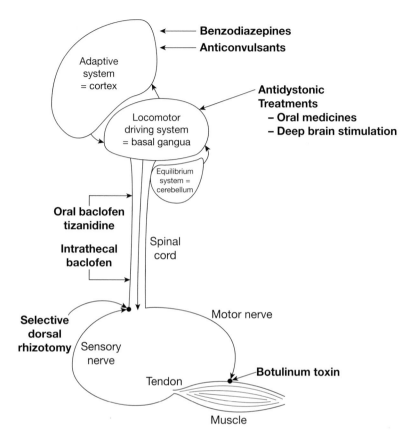

Figure 6.1. Medical movement therapies and where they work.

MUSCLE RELAXANTS
These relax all the muscles in the body from your forehead to your little toe. They also work on both sides equally, so side effects are often seen before any benefit. However, they can be very useful if there are painful spasms.

Baclofen has been used since the 1970s. It reduces the excitability of the motor nerves coming out from the spine. However, it is not easily transported in the body to the areas where it works, and therefore big doses of oral medicine may be necessary to allow any muscle relaxation. As such, it has a narrow *therapeutic window*, i.e. if the dose is increased only a little beyond that required to achieve the desired effect it can cause significant side effects of floppiness and sleepiness.

Diazepam is extremely effective but highly sedating, and the body gets used to it, so it stops working if it is used too much. It can be useful after surgery or to reduce muscle cramps at night.

The next two are used very rarely in hemiplegia, but knowledge of them is important

Tizanidine has been around since the late 1990s, and we know a lot about it in adults but very little in children. It is thought that it causes less sleepiness.

Dantrolene works directly at the muscle level. It can be very effective but has marked side effects of weakness and, catastrophically, liver failure in around 1% of patients. I do not prescribe it personally.

ANTIDYSTONIC AGENTS

A predominantly dystonic problem, where the muscle tone fluctuates, is seen much more rarely than one where the muscle tone is generally high. If, however, the predominant motor difficulty in a child is a dystonic hemiplegia, then we can try to improve the fluidity of movement using medicines developed for adult conditions in which the basal ganglia stop working, such as Parkinson or Huntington disease. The basal ganglia work like a ring road for the brain. All the information going in and all the messages coming out need to travel along it. When there is damage to the basal ganglia, it is equivalent to trying to get all the traffic into and out of a city through one junction – impossible during rush hour but remarkably manageable in the middle of the night.

What we are trying to do with antidystonic agents is to provide more of the natural chemicals that work at the basal ganglia level. This is not a magic cure but it does help the individual to make the most of the fluidity of their motor control. To continue the ring road concept above, we cannot open up extra junctions but we can widen the road and put in a rolling speed limit. By doing this, subtle but significant improvements in motor control can be achieved, including less abnormal posturing of the limbs, reduced painful spasms, and easier reach and use of the hand.

As antidystonic agents do not cause weakness or sleepiness but work on selective movements, a trial of one to see if it helps or not is sensible in children with dystonic hemiplegia. Generally children should be started on such treatment only by specialist units.

Trihexyphenidyl is probably the medicine with the greatest potential. This anticholinergic agent works at the level of the basal ganglia, and its side effects come from its mode of action:

- Constipation – it relaxes the bowel.
- Urinary retention – it relaxes the bladder, which results in less frequent urination of bigger volumes. It does not have any effect on the kidneys.
- Excessively dry mouth and, more rarely, irritability, sleep problems or a reactive increase in abnormal movements.

All side effects are reversible when the medicine is stopped.

Other medicines could be considered including **dopamine** (a *neurotransmitter* – transmits messages from neurons) and **tetrabenazine**. Their side effects tend to be more marked, and often finding the right medicine for a child is a process of trial and error.

Some anticonvulsants, such as **carbamazepine** and **levetiracetam**, also help with movement effect – so much so that there are several international trials looking at their use in movement disorders alone.

Focal (targeted) medical and surgical interventions

BOTULINUM TOXIN A INJECTIONS
Botulinum toxin type A was first used in cerebral palsy in the mid-1990s. It is licensed for use in children over the age of two years with dynamic equinus foot deformity caused by spasticity in ambulant (i.e. the children are able to walk) cerebral palsy – including hemiplegia. However, a great deal of research has looked at injections into other muscles and glands that cause local functional difficulty, including multilevel lower- and upper-limb use.

- Scope, the national organization for people with cerebral palsy, called it the most significant step forward in management for 50 years.
- The American Academy of Neurology has stated that it should be universally offered as a treatment option in childhood movement disorders.

Any joint has a big *agonist* muscle (i.e. the one primarily responsible for movement, e.g. the biceps at the elbow) and a smaller *antagonist* muscle (i.e. the one working in opposition, e.g. the triceps on the other side). When the muscles are activated the big muscle predominates and pulls the joint out of a functional position. The treatment theory behind botulinum toxin A is that it works to relax the agonist and strengthen the antagonist.

Evidence-based guidelines on the use of botulinum toxin are regularly updated, with the most recent being the European Consensus Statement 2009. This focuses on medicolegal and medico-economic factors (i.e. the legal and economic aspects of its use), common indications and how to obtain the best benefit, appropriate assessment, what areas for injections are accepted as appropriate, dosage, safety, administration, re-evaluation, when to repeat and when to stop. Anyone involved in assessment for injection should be aware of these guidelines.

Botulinum toxins are naturally made by a bacterium called *Clostridium botulinum*. Type A is the most effective. It works by specifically targeting the junction between the nerve and the muscle – the *motor end plate*. It irreversibly blocks the message getting through, allowing the overactivated muscle to relax and stretch. The motor end plate shrivels up to the point where the fatty sheath ends; after a short period, a new junction starts to grow. This means that the direct effect lasts for around three months. However, the pulse of stretch and relaxation in the muscle generally results in benefits that can last up to a year.

On the positive side, this means that the position of the limb at joints can become more normal, and the muscles can stretch and grow in unison with the underlying bone. On the negative side, it temporarily weakens the injected muscle further. Again, that balance of strength and stretch.

Botulinum toxin injections can be very useful in managing painful spasms.

Multidisciplinary assessment of muscle tightness, weakness, function and dysfunction is, once again, the key to whether it will be helpful or not. Here, an ounce of experience is worth a ton of theory; sometimes it is as important *not* to use injections as it may be to use them at other times. Although any doctor in the UK is licensed to use botulinum toxin, you would be advised to seek out a specialist centre where you will receive specialist advice on whether or not this treatment would be appropriate for your child.

The injections themselves are generally given with some sedation or local anaesthetic in a hospital day care unit. Occasionally a general anaesthetic is used. It is also very important to inject the right muscle, so the use of muscle stimulators or direct ultrasound guidance to check needle placement is increasingly accepted as best clinical practice.

It is also not a treatment to be used without the involvement of local physiotherapists and occupational therapists. Your child may not need any increase in therapy, but a re-evaluation of the management plan is vital. The Association of Paediatric Chartered Physiotherapists (APCP) has provided careful guidance on what is and is not appropriate.

FUNCTIONAL ELECTRICAL STIMULATION
The theory behind this is to stimulate the antagonist muscles directly. Electrical pads providing a low current are placed over muscles in the child's arm or leg and switched on. Trials show short-lived strengthening but no long-term benefit.

ORTHOPAEDIC SURGERY
Surgery is required when any deformity in the muscles and tendons leads to fixed tightness across joints that, in turn, leads to functional difficulties for the child. Any abnormal position in a child with hemiplegia is even more obvious as a result of comparison with the other side.

The most common orthopaedic problems seen in hemiplegia

Arm
- Flexion at the elbow
- Flexion at the wrist and fingers
- Thumb stuck across and in the palm

Leg
- Tiptoe position at the ankle (*equinus*)
- In-turning at the ankle (*varus foot*)
- Out-turning at the ankle (*valgus*)
- Flexion at the knee
- Less frequently, internal rotation at the hip

Generally, the surgical options are to

- lengthen short muscles and tendons;
- move the awkward pull of overactive muscles;
- provide a stable base for walking by manipulating bones in the foot;
- untwist other bones.

Nowadays surgeons try to do as much as required in a single operation (*multilevel surgery*) and then provide early active rehabilitation. This minimizes weakness and maximizes outcome. Timing of any intervention is vital, and the orthopaedic team will provide guidance on this. Obviously, the child should be better off in the long term, having had surgery, than he or she would have been without it.

Arm surgery
The goals are to improve grasp, release and reach and also the appearance of the arm and hand. Thumb, finger, wrist and elbow deformities may also be assessed and treated in this way.

Muscle and tendon lengthening and *split transfers* are the most frequent procedures, with bone manipulation used more rarely. Muscle lengthening keeps the most power, and in split transfer procedures the tendon is attached to the opposite side of the bone in order to bring the position of the limb into balance. Specific post-operative care is important for a good outcome, with the use of casts or strengthening programmes supervised by other members of the multidisciplinary team.

Leg surgery
Equinus describes a walking position up on the toes, similar to that of a ballet dancer performing, a sprinter running or someone wearing high heels. In hemiplegia this causes a relative misalignment of the limb, imbalance at the hip and a flexible curve of the spine. Some equinus can compensate in part for the slight difference in leg length generally seen in hemiplegia (up to 1.5 centimetres being normal).

Careful assessment is required, and the correct timing of any procedure depends on the individual child. If function is delayed or lost, then it is appropriate to intervene. Operative management of any contracture can either be lengthening of the Achilles tendon (triple-cut elongation of the Achilles tendon, which attaches the calf muscles to the heel bone) or physical stretching of the muscles involved (*gastrocnemius slide*). More strength is maintained using a muscle approach, which is important as 50% of all power in walking is generated by these muscles. Overlengthening is far worse from a biomechanical point of view than underlengthening, as the former can make it very difficult to walk. 'Whatever is worth doing is not worth overdoing.'

If the foot is deformed because of abnormal muscle pull, then it is also important that the child has surgery at the appropriate time. If surgery is delayed, skeletal changes can worsen and the base of walking and standing is made even more precarious. It is also very painful to bear weight through the wrong part of the foot. In studies, over one-third (38%) of children with hemiplegia developed an in-turning – varus – deformity – whereas fewer than 2% progressed to a flat footed out-turning – valgus – deformity.

In **varus deformity**, initially a split tendon transfer of the muscle pulling in may be enough (*posterior tibialis tendon transfer*). At a later stage, bone surgery to the ankle and foot may become necessary. In a **valgus deformity**, however, fixation of the structures of the foot is necessary.

If **knee flexion** is causing a functional problem, then hamstring (one of the long muscles at the back of the thigh) muscle lengthening may be necessary. This allows more movement in the knee joint. However, the capsule at the back of the knee is where all the blood vessels and nerves for the lower leg pass through. So it is vital not to put too much strain on them and, once again, overlengthen. Extra range can be gained slowly in a controlled fashion by surgically stapling the front of the long bone growth plate (*femoral epiphysis*) just above the knee. Continued slow bony growth at the back can straighten the apparent position of the knee over a period of years, and at the right time the staples can be removed.

Sometimes it may also be relevant to correct excessive twisting of the upper thigh bone or femur (internal rotation). Careful consideration of what is going on throughout the whole of the lower leg is necessary to prevent the deformity switching the other way after any intervention.

Even more invasive interventions
Parents often ask about these at clinics, so although they are generally of little relevance in hemiplegia, I will cover them briefly.

INTRATHECAL BACLOFEN
To overcome the problems with peripheral side effects such as sleepiness, when given orally, the muscle relaxant baclofen can be injected directly to the space surrounding the spinal cord. To do this an *indwelling epidural catheter* is placed through a spinal disc and tunnelled under the skin to the front of the abdomen (stomach). A small reservoir (about 7.5 centimetres diameter) for the baclofen, with a tiny computer on the side, is placed under the stomach muscles and attached to the tube. Top-ups, injected into the reservoir, are necessary every few months, using a local anaesthetic and an ultrasound

scanner to guide the needle. Flow rates can be altered using an external computer that communicates directly with the one on the reservoir. Batteries need to be changed every six years.

Intrathecal baclofen is most frequently used to help children with severe cerebral palsy affecting all their limbs. There are a few case reports of it being used in children with hemiplegia.

SELECTIVE DORSAL RHIZOTOMY
This type of surgery interrupts the overactive spinal messages by irreversibly cutting some of the tiny nerves going into the spine, so reducing muscle tone in specific muscle groups. Weakness is increased, side effects are marked and its use in hemiplegia is anecdotal; certainly, nothing is reported in the medical literature.

DEEP BRAIN STIMULATION
A few children with a severe pure dystonic hemiplegia have had this intervention. The muscle tone must be fluctuating, without any degree of underlying weakness or tightness. A device similar to a pacemaker is inserted directly into certain specific areas of the basal ganglia. This stimulates the brain directly to try to organize the signals in the motor system.

The insertion of this 'brain pacemaker' has led to an improvement on dystonia rating scales of between 5% and 20%, as well as in general quality of life in movement disorders as a whole; however, there is no specific information about the likely outcome in hemiplegia.

Alternative and complementary treatments
Many types of complementary or alternative treatment are used internationally in the management of movement disorders, such as hemiplegia, in children. Some have been found to be very beneficial in individual cases, although there are very few good-quality studies showing long-term benefit. Generally, there is little good scientific evidence for most complementary therapies. But equally there have been very few properly conducted studies of standard treatments for hemiplegia, and as parents hope against hope that a cure will be found for their child, many people are attracted by alternative options.

However, although most practitioners are dedicated, careful and holistic in their approach, without proper regulation there is the potential for malpractice and considerable expense to the family. Properly conducted clinical trials (such as the one recently completed for cranial osteopathy for children with cerebral palsy) and the development of regulatory bodies are both vital. Without these, as open-minded advocates, we have to remain open yet guarded to the claims of such therapeutic options.

The most common complementary therapies include those listed below, with the reasoning behind them and comment on governance.

Acupuncture A reduction in high muscle tone following the use of both acupuncture and acupressure has been observed in children with spastic cerebral palsy. The degree of benefit is very individual, but the evidence from several case series (series of case studies) is encouraging.

Alexander technique A method of 'physical and mental re-education' in which the focus is on inducing core stability with 'self-improvement' techniques.

Amino acid therapy All the vogue in the 1990s. Extremely high doses of oral amino acids are combined with patterning physiotherapy. The latter provides short-term benefit. The former is at best physiologically questionable.

Aromatherapy The use of volatile essential plant oils and aromatic compounds to relax overactive muscle contraction.

Bowen technique Specialist osteopathic massage of muscles and *fascia* (the sheaths around bundles of muscle fibres) claiming to improve movement and posture.

Chinese herbal medicine Claims to work by altering the balance of muscle tone using traditional herbal approaches. Limited evidence base but some anecdotal benefit.

Cranial osteopathy This is the treatment of musculoskeletal problems by inducing self-recovery. Gentle manipulation of the head provides a balance within the whole body. A very impressive multicentre trial has recently been completed on its use in cerebral palsy as a whole, without clinically significant benefit. A number of case series do show consistent improvement in posture, range of movement and comfort, especially in babies, but longer-term benefits are far less obvious.

Chiropractic therapy Skilled manipulation, especially of the spine, claiming to improve the function of joints and surrounding soft tissues.

Hippotherapy Specifically uses the movement of the horse or pony as a means of treatment, rather than teaching riding skills. The child's balance adapts to the horse's movement, improving posture and coordination and reducing muscle spasm. There are encouraging case series that report improvement in core stability in children with bilateral (two-sided) cerebral palsy but less in children with hemiplegia.

Homeopathy, including specific 'G therapy' of tissue salts and herb extracts, is said to be useful for a variety of neurodevelopmental disorders including cerebral palsy, but the clinical evidence base is limited.

Hyperbaric oxygen therapy The theory is to heal damaged tissue in the central nervous system by removing free radicals, using high oxygen concentrations in pressure chambers. Benefit has been shown if used in the acute phase following injury but long-term and non-acute usage is questionable at best.

Reflexology Pressure application to the feet and hands, with claims to restore equilibrium.

Scotson technique Focuses on strengthening of the diaphragm, the theory being to improve oxygen flow to the damaged brain by gentle 'manual delivery' of breath and pulse-like pressures.

Suit/Adeli/Thera/Spider therapy Uses repetitive patterning exercises in a tight-fitting suit that provides resistance to movement. The suit is connected by hooks, rings and elastic bungee cords to provide adjustable pressure and support at different joint levels. It is claimed to improve motor development and decrease bone demineralization. Many of my patients' parents have found the results encouraging, although it is physically tiring for the child and there have been only short-term improvements noted.

Yoga and **Pilates** Various different types of physical and breathing exercises, sometimes linked to meditation, to aid relaxation, strengthen, improve balance and reduce stiffness.

Stem cell therapy
We are all made up of many different cell types. There is no point in taking some 'differentiated' (specialized) liver cells, putting them into the heart, and expecting them to beat. However, very early indeed in our development, as described in Chapter 2, we create cell lines that have not yet differentiated – *pluripotential stem cells*. Some of these basic building blocks are maintained into later life in areas such as the umbilical cord or even in bone marrow. The theory is that putting these stem cells back into parts of the body that are not working may, in time, lead to regeneration of the lost function as the stem cells differentiate into (become specialized like) the cell types around them.

Unfortunately, as yet, there is no reliable medical evidence of short-, mid- or long-term benefit, in spite of numerous impressive individual case reports, particularly when using the patient's own harvested umbilical cord stem cells. As advocates, we have to be careful not to be carried away by sensational claims, no matter how desperate we are for a cure. The potential miracles have to be balanced by the potential side effects that have been observed: epilepsy, infection, and worsening of disability. Without such careful review and clear evidence from clinical trials, there is certainly no possibility of widespread acceptance in mainstream medical practice at present.

Anti-epileptic interventions
When you treat epilepsy you have to juggle three things to get the best individual treatment plan:

- the frequency, duration and impact of the seizures themselves,
- how the individual is developing in all areas in the times between seizures, and
- the potential side effects of the medicines you are using.

Treatment of epilepsy associated with hemiplegia is in many ways no different from epilepsy as a whole, although it can be difficult to gain complete control with medicines. As we have seen, learning and behaviour can be affected even more, so it is important to bear this in mind when deciding which anticonvulsants are relevant, so as not to make the third factor overwhelming.

MEDICAL INTERVENTIONS

Most seizures have a local origin in the areas of brain that are damaged. First-line medicines for treatment of this type of epilepsy are

- carbamazepine,
- sodium valproate, and
- lamotrigine.

Topiramate can also be useful, but it has higher rates of behavioural problems associated with it.

Other medicines can be used in combination therapy: levetiracetam is particularly useful when there are structural problems in the brain. Vigabatrin is too, but careful review of vision is necessary as there is a risk of non-reversible visual field defects. A child should rarely be taking more than two anticonvulsants at any one time – any more and the side effects are likely to outweigh any benefit. Control can be difficult, and is often impossible, and the emphasis should be on minimizing the frequency and duration of events and gaining the best quality of life without overwhelming drug side effects such as sleepiness and learning and behavioural difficulties.

Other medical options are needed with specific patterns of epilepsy. In infants and very young children, the use of high-dose steroids may be necessary to dampen down very complicated seizures. Following a *ketogenic diet*, i.e. one high in fats and low in carbohydrates, with the support of specialist teams, can also help by switching the metabolism of the brain from sugars and starches to fats.

An emergency treatment protocol may also be necessary, with advice about what medicine to give, what to do and when to call for help when a seizure has started. A family of drugs called the benzodiazepines are used: midazolam in the cheek, lorazepam under the tongue or diazepam rectally.

SURGICAL INTERVENTIONS

As the seizures are generally driven by one area, a surgical approach to treatment is sometimes considered in cases of 'refractory or intractable epilepsy' (uncontrolled with medicines).

The two main approaches are

- **vagal nerve stimulation** – an electrical stimulator wrapped around one of the major nerves to and from the brain, and
- either electrical or physical removal of the part of the brain driving the epilepsy – **lobectomy** or **hemispherectomy**.

One condition associated with hemiplegia – Sturge–Weber syndrome, in which abnormal blood vessels on one side of the face are mirrored by abnormal blood vessels in the brain – is generally treated by surgical excision as the rates of intractable epilepsy are very high.

Obviously, consideration of surgical approaches is not to be taken lightly. Specialist national centres with large teams of experts, including paediatric neurologists, electrophysiologists and neurosurgeons, are necessary to assess, discuss and carry out any procedure.

Language assessments and interventions

Although some children with congenital hemiplegia have developmental language disorders, the plasticity of the brain means that communication is generally well preserved, though at the expense of other skills such as visuospatial perception. Early left-sided injury can lead to subtle problems with verbal structure and comprehension, but those with injury on the right side show no difference in these areas from the population as a whole. However, some studies show that the level of difficulty with left-sided injury may be related to overall learning ability.

Acquired hemiplegia leads more frequently to acquired language problems. Following the initial damage or injury that leads to hemiplegia, communication problems are relatively common. Most are temporary, but some difficulties can persist, especially difficulties in expressing oneself. *Aphasia*, a lack of, or *dysphasia*, a difficulty in, understanding and expression of speech occurs when any damage to the brain also includes the language areas.

The capacity of the brain to recover depends on the age at which the hemiplegia is acquired, the site and size of the damage and, once again, whether the child also has seizures. Damage after around the age of eight years in the left cerebral cortex generally leads to prolonged word-finding and word-processing problems. Children with both a left-sided cerebral problem (i.e. right hemiplegia) and seizures are most likely, unfortunately, to have the greatest difficulties.

The speech and language therapist is vital to assess the child, provide appropriate communication aids, and liaise with parents, carers and other members of the multidisciplinary team regarding coping strategies. Again, regular reappraisal of any management plan is necessary. Direct therapy to optimize speech relies on exercises to improve speech production. Alternative approaches may involve teaching strategies to compensate for any area of difficulty. Treatment can also address problems with indirect language skills, such as attention and listening abilities.

Intervention in emotional and behavioural disorders

Psychology and child and adolescent mental health services are vital in supporting local community services in the management of behavioural difficulties in children with hemiplegia. To reiterate, the problems most frequently seen are these:

- anxiety,
- challenging behaviour or 'conduct disorders', including irritability and disruptive behaviour,
- inattention,
- autistic spectrum disorders, and
- secondary reactive problems, including depression; obsessive–compulsive traits; anorexia nervosa.

Firstly, one of the most basic interventions in managing emotional and behavioural difficulties in children with hemiplegia is helping parents to see that such problems are not a reflection on their parenting skills but a result of the underlying brain disorder. Although this explains the situation, it does not mean that we should accept the problem and not actively treat it.

Secondly, the presence of seizures and the side effects of any medication used in their management can have a direct effect on behaviour. Improving control of the epilepsy or a change of anticonvulsants can bring about a dramatic improvement in behaviour. Topiramate, sodium valproate and vigabatrin, in particular, can cause difficulties.

Thirdly, it is important to acknowledge the effect of disability on self-esteem and self-image and the relevance of that to psychological well-being. While taking these factors into account, emotional and behavioural problems should be approached in the same way as with any other child. A focus on maintaining consistency in any treatment programme across all social situations, including home and school, is the keystone for any treatment programme.

Anxiety
The treatment for specific phobias is desensitization, through encouragement and initial exposure to things related to but not the explicit fear itself. The skill is in engaging the child and using sufficient stepping stones from a non-threatening exposure all the way up to the thing most feared itself, without provoking anything more than mild anxiety. As we said earlier, separation anxiety is one of the major problems, and this is dealt with in a similar way, with longer and longer periods of parting.

Various other techniques to relax and reassure can be taught, especially to children who are slightly older. Often, anxiety can be significantly reduced by giving advance warning and avoiding surprises.

Challenging behaviour
Controlling and containing children who are oppositional, defiant and even aggressive to themselves and others can be a huge challenge and requires endless patience. Additional support for the parents and classroom support staff is vital. The usual approach is to reward good behaviour and ignore bad.

Fair, firm, consistent boundaries are necessary, with bucketloads of praise, not just for doing things but also for just 'being', helping the child to reflect on his or her own feelings. Having a brief non-threatening 'time out' is often necessary to allow the child to calm down. Occasionally it may be necessary to avoid some obvious causes of stress, particularly in the early stages of management. Unrecognized learning difficulties may also be a significant factor in some children.

Focus on a few key areas to work on and don't expect your child to be perfect. Common sense is a wonderful thing, but it is hard to maintain when faced with real defiance from a child.

Inattention
Once any epilepsy has been treated, possible psychotherapeutic programmes are the key to management. These focus on presenting tasks in sufficiently small sections and providing frequent repetition until the child can cope. It is also important to avoid excessive criticism.

Occasionally, if the inattention and hyperactivity is extreme, medicines such as methylphenidate or dexamfetamine are used. These are stimulant drugs of the brain that work by increasing the capacity to concentrate. They should be used only as part of a comprehensive treatment programme, as the potential side effects of restlessness, sleeplessness, headaches and confusion are all significant.

Autistic spectrum disorders
In their most severe forms, autistic spectrum disorders (ASD) are comparatively rare. Improvement is rarely dramatic and behavioural modification can be difficult. Consistent patience is vital. There are a multitude of targeted approaches to management, but the starting points are a careful structured assessment of autistic symptoms and an age- and developmental level-appropriate psychological evaluation of learning. From there, individual intervention programmes are set up, reviewed on a regular basis and continued in the long term. Problems are likely to be life long. Milder forms of ASD, such as Asperger syndrome, may be more common and recognition is important in order to understand and make allowances for a child's behaviour. Obsessive–compulsive traits are also seen more frequently.

Secondary reactive difficulties
Depression, withdrawal, difficulties in forming close relationships and anorexia nervosa are all more common in children and young people with hemiplegia than their classmates, and particularly at adolescence. Again, these may be associated with factors such as epilepsy, learning difficulties and ASD. Treatment programmes are based on individual support and social and self-help skills. Therapy and medication may be effective in some severely depressed teenagers.

Problems as an adolescent and adult

All clinical problems in hemiplegia remain life long. Learning and emotional difficulties, both directly and indirectly related to the hemiplegia and epilepsy, are the most significant factors in independent living as an adult.

The patient treatment pathway becomes rockiest at the time when young people are feeling most insecure, namely when independence from home and school looms. This is not helped by the clinical network that they have experienced as a child seeming to disappear from under their feet. A lack of support can amplify the sense of anxiety to a great degree. With guidance from patient advocacy groups such as HemiHelp, health and education services are trying to focus on this period with transitional planning (see Chapters 8 and 9). The problem is finding a service to transit to: adult services, apart from general practice, tend to be much less holistic and multidisciplinary than children's services in their approach.

With regard to movement difficulties, the most significant changes in the long term are increasing pain and fatigue, particularly in the affected leg. Careful assessment of muscle power in adults with hemiplegia shows a reduced muscle volume of up to 50% in comparison with the population as a whole. This means that, as people with hemiplegia get older, there is less muscle reserve to help keep them moving. It is likely, however, that early muscle strengthening programmes may help the individual maintain power levels significantly higher than this.

With increasing independence, reliance on adult support for two-handed tasks in many activities of daily living becomes increasingly impractical. Strategies need to be worked on early enough to genuinely help the individual and appropriate equipment sought out.

Learning, emotional and behavioural support and seizure management need to be continued with regular reassessment and reflection. I know far too many young people who started taking medicines as a child but have had no review of their treatments since and just carry on taking the same prescription.

Universal provision of appropriate support for adults with hemiplegia, or any disability come to that, should be, and is, becoming a priority for health services.

Summary
- The patient pathway:
  - the team around the child – child- and family-centred services;
  - multidisciplinary working – best practice is the team approach.
- Assessments:
  - movement – observation, evaluation and re-evaluation of developmental progress over time/treatment;

- ○ other developmental factors may also be necessary such as visual, visuospatial, communication and psychology assessments.
- Investigations may be relevant and include:
  - ○ brain scans,
  - ○ blood tests, and
  - ○ electrical scans, if there is a history of possible seizures.
- Interventions in hemiplegia:
  - ○ motor:
    - – therapy services focus on function and activity, support and education;
    - – medical treatments aim to slow the rate of secondary deformity and relieve symptoms; they can be focal or generalized in nature;
    - – surgical options aim to minimize deformity.
    - – alternative/complementary therapies;
    - – stem cell treatment;
  - ○ epilepsy management and anticonvulsants;
  - ○ communication programmes for specific language difficulties, and social communication difficulties;
  - ○ emotional and behavioural problems, of which the major ones encountered are
    - – anxiety,
    - – challenging behaviour,
    - – hyperactivity and inattention,
    - – autistic spectrum disorders, and
    - – reactive responses to disability.
- Adult health service provision.

Chapter 7
Family life

Liz Barnes

Early years

As you read this, you could find yourself thinking of your child with hemiplegia as just a bundle of problems to be solved, and life as a never-ending series of hurdles to get over, many of them involving mysterious sets of initials: CDC, OT, DLA, SEN, IEP. But your child is a child like any other and a member of a family, and family life needs to go on. And it will.

> *Take things one day at a time and celebrate what your child can do, not what they can't do.*

> *Give yourself the space to 'grieve' and slowly realize that your child will have a life, it will just be different from the one you visualized for her.*

If this is your first child, you will probably not have any firm ideas of what to expect, and it may be easier to accept your child perhaps taking longer to reach the usual 'milestones' – sitting, walking, toilet training, and so on. If you have an older child or children it will be more difficult to avoid comparisons. In either case it does not help that no-one can tell you how your child will progress. HemiHelp asked its members what advice they would give parents setting out on life with a child with hemiplegia. There were 518 answers, many of them repeating simple phrases such as 'Don't panic', 'Take each day as it comes' and 'You are not alone', and you will find others quoted throughout this chapter.

In your child's first years, life will be dominated by hospital and child development centre/unit appointments of one kind or another, and some children with hemiplegia will develop epilepsy or have other associated conditions that affect their general development. But most children with hemiplegia will be developing in line with others of the same age in many ways – smiling, sitting, playing and feeding themselves using their non-affected hand/arm, beginning to talk – so there will be achievements to celebrate. Most of them also learn to walk without too much difficulty, although perhaps a little later than average (and they will need physiotherapy and possibly other treatment to correct their gait). The main focus at this time will be to try to develop the child's use of his or her affected hand and arm. The whole family will become sick of the words 'Use both hands, please' (I often thought of making a tape with the words repeated over and over). Your physiotherapist will probably give you exercises to do between visits, but it will be more fun if you also use play to encourage your child to stretch and use his or her weaker hand. Get the whole family involved. HemiHelp has a DVD of exercises you can do at home, and an information sheet with ideas for toys and activities to try.

> Make exercises fun and part of daily routine like teeth brushing.

> We tried to do everything the physiotherapist told us but made it all lots of fun (and something he USUALLY! wanted to do). We feel this has given B the best start physically.

> The occupational therapist can also give advice on play, and local toy libraries are a great place to try things out.

> Take them to a mums and tots group, swimming – don't isolate yourself and your child.

Getting out with your child is also important. Activities outside the home can combine fun and exercise with the chance to mix with other children. In the first year or two this could be a parent and toddler group, one o'clock club or baby swimming, and later a playgroup or other pre-school setting. It is best if these can be close to home, so that friendships started in the group can be easily continued outside it, and it will make going up to school easier if children your child already knows are going too. And these are also good places for parents to make friends who they will be able to turn to for support in the years to come.

What all this boils down to is that your young child's life should be as normal as possible. Parents can become so anxious about their children's progress that they spend all their time ferrying them to one therapy after another, which is not just exhausting for everyone but leaves little time or energy for normal family life. And, while stretching and strengthening the weaker side is important, in the end the child will find his or her own way around challenges as they arise, whether that means using one or both hands.

> By treating your child as normally as possible you give them a good chance at leading a very normal life. Focus on can not can't, and encourage them to try things.

> M has found ways of doing things on his own like holding certain things, cutting paper, etc., and I'm sure he will continue to adapt to things throughout his life.

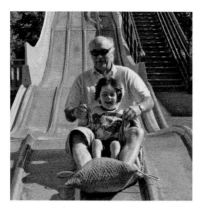

Don't wrap your child in cotton wool. Make them 'get on with it', they'll thank you for it later in life. (Adult with hemiplegia)

The young child should also be encouraged to become as independent as possible with washing, toileting and dressing. This is another area in which the occupational therapist will be able to help with advice, and HemiHelp and Scope have information sheets that can be downloaded.

With dressing, for example, there are some simple guidelines to follow: clothes should be loose, tops should open at the front with Velcro fastenings or have loose necks (put over head, then affected arm in first), trousers and skirts should have elastic waists. Shoes should also fasten with Velcro or with curly laces (and, believe it or not, you can lace shoes one-handed!).

Five to eleven
Once they are at school, children often get less physiotherapy and occupational therapy, although if they go to a special school there will be therapists on the staff, and in mainstream regular therapy may be written into a Statement of Special Educational Needs if they have one. (If possible, the occupational therapist should also visit the school to make an assessment and advise staff of the child's needs in the classroom – positioning, seating, writing aids, etc.)

So it falls more to the family to keep them exercising – or perhaps active might be a better word here, because they will be less and less willing to do anything that smacks of therapy. Fortunately, during the primary school years children with hemiplegia can keep up with their classmates in many activities. Many can play football quite well, for example, although unfortunately this is often seen as strictly a boys' sport.

Most children with hemiplegia can learn to swim and cycle – two skills that will not only help keep them fit and strengthen their muscles, but will also make it easier for them to mix with others of their age. Some may continue to need stabilizers or prefer a three-wheeled bike (it may be possible to get a specialized bike through occupational therapy or a charity – see links below).

My daughter can't ride a bike, so we bought her a go-cart which she uses to exercise her legs.

B likes going out as a family on our bikes. As she is unable to ride a bike on her own we have a tandem.

Young children are very accepting of one another, and do not pay much attention to the fact that someone has a weak arm or a limp, but as they grow older – usually some time during junior school – they become more aware of differences. So the child with hemiplegia will realize that he or she finds some things more difficult than classmates do, or someone may make a spiteful remark about a splint or call him or her a name. Families with a child with hemiplegia are scattered around the country, and most children are in mainstream schools, so they may never meet another person like them. So, if other children tease or bully they can feel very alone.

Parents also need to watch out for any changes in their child's behaviour or emotional state; this might reflect difficulties at school or with his or her friendship group. Previously undetected specific learning difficulties may be emerging – problems with literacy and numeracy are quite common in children with hemiplegia – so parents should keep in touch with the school to make sure their son or daughter is getting appropriate support. Also, Dr Carole Yude's work on friendship and popularity in mainstream primary schools* showed that children with hemiplegia had more than average difficulty making and keeping friends, and that it was the more subtle, less visible problems associated with hemiplegia, such as low self-confidence, immaturity and vulnerability, which seemed to be responsible rather than the physical disability alone.

All this is why it can be useful to make contact with other families through HemiHelp or other disability networks. Parents who come to fun and activity days always remark on their child's relief on finding there are other children like her or him. And indeed adults: a HemiHelp trustee with hemiplegia was helping out at one such event, and noticed children pointing at her: 'Oh, look, she has it too!'

Of course activity days – whether for sports, crafts, music or drama – do not just allow children to meet other people with hemiplegia. Their main aim is to give them a taster of things that they may never have thought of trying, or may have been put off because other children might laugh at their efforts. Finding a sport or other activity that they enjoy will not only exercise their body but boost their confidence. We can also hope that extensive media coverage of the Paralympic Games, at which British athletes with hemiplegia and other types of cerebral palsy have been winning lots of medals for swimming and cycling, will have raised the profile of disability sport in the UK for the next generation.

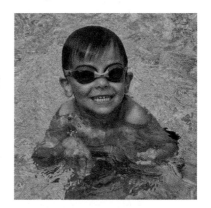

The HemiHelp survey showed that children were already involved in an amazing range of activities, including football, swimming, cycling, sailing, dance, drama, music, tennis, table tennis, martial arts, gymnastics, trampolining and horse riding –

---

*   See HemiHelp information sheet 'Friendship and Popularity in Mainstream Primary Schools' some in disabled settings but many at least partly in mainstream. Some of course prefer quieter pursuits such as chess, reading and computer games. Many children are also members of youth organizations such as Brownies, Cubs, Woodcraft Folk, etc. And, of course, all these activities are also opportunities to make new friends.

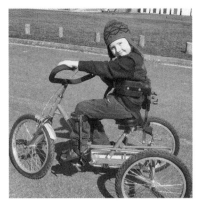

> *Give them opportunities to do things even if you know that they will only achieve a little. We took S to a climbing wall when he was about six because he desperately wanted to have a go. The instructor was great. He got about three feet off the ground but thought it was marvellous and still talks about the experience.*

> *D took up squash after a HemiHelp fun day, which he now plays at a local club and as part of a school team. He also played tennis for the first time at a fun day, which gave him confidence to play at his secondary school too.*

Of course life is not all about fun and games. Treating children with hemiplegia as normally as possible also means that they should help with the chores like everyone else. Allowances need to be made for their abilities, but they should be encouraged to learn new skills and use their ingenuity to get round challenges. Simple aids such as non-slip mats and spiked chopping boards to hold cheese, fruit or vegetables for slicing can make helping with cooking easier, for example.

This is the age at which families do the most things together – holidays, days out, outdoor activities – when children are old enough to take part but not too old to want to do them independently. Having a child with hemiplegia in the family can make this more complicated – he or she probably cannot walk as far, gets tired more easily, and so on. Many families reported their frustration at this, but others have been able to make the most of activities together.

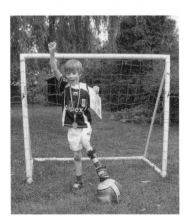

> *We do tend to do activities that would be beneficial to him. Days out tend to be planned with less walking, frequent stops, etc. Holidays are to places that he would enjoy.*

> *We now have a disabled parking badge for him which is a great help on days out, etc. We ensure that we can include him in all that we do and encourage him to join in.*

> *We get along just fine with T in the family. We all look after him and we go camping, swimming and day tripping together. He is the centre of our family life but in a good way.*

If your child has complex needs that limit activity as
a family, short breaks (also known as respite care), whether community-based or
residential, provide opportunities for disabled children to have enjoyable experiences
that help them become more independent and form friendships outside their family. At
the same time their families get a regular break from the demands of caring for a
disabled child. Or you may as a parent feel the need for a break from time to time. Local
authorities have a duty to provide a short breaks service to disabled children and their
carers; contact them to see what it can offer, or see the links at the end of the chapter for
charities that provide this service.

Eleven to sixteen

In other words: puberty, adolescence, teens. This
is a trying time for every family, but, here again,
the usual headaches are likely to be magnified. Secondary school is a more stressful
environment than primary, and the other students more likely to bully or tease. This
stress may show up as greater anxiety or irritability at home (which can also be caused
by just plain tiredness).

As physical appearance (one's own and others') becomes more important, looking
different, wearing special shoes or a splint, or appearing clumsy can all affect the young
person's sense of confidence. For girls in particular, and at this age girls develop earlier
than boys, growing up brings new challenges. Finding suitable shoes that are also
fashionable, putting on make-up and jewellery, doing their hair in the latest styles – these
are all challenges to be overcome (see HemiHelp's one-handed tips sheet for ideas).

At this time family support is more crucial than ever. Parents should give
encouragement with schoolwork but also find time to relax with activities that the
young person enjoys, whether this means continuing with those that he or she is already
involved in or finding new interests – possibly through after-school clubs. Many
HemiHelp members' children of this age have graduated from Cubs and Brownies to
Scouts and Guides; some are doing a Duke of Edinburgh's Award. Other new interests
include snooker, tenpin bowling, badminton, squash, golf, photography and film-

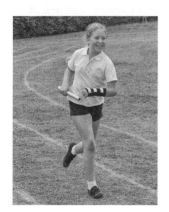

making, as well as volunteering – for example helping to
run a group for younger children. And again, taking part in
these activities can help young people make new friends.

*Scouts has been fantastic – disability no problem, safe/structured
environment. He has just been to Germany for six nights and is
going on a five-night watersports course in May half-term.
Scouts has helped in so many ways – especially self-confidence.*

*I was told R may never walk but he plays football for England
and has been around the world.*

Guides, help at Brownies, book club, plays tenor horn in a band.

It must, however, be said that when it comes to competitive sports, at this stage it becomes more difficult to keep up with other young people of the same age. Depending to some extent on where you live, there may be opportunities to continue to develop and compete in a disabled setting, but some young people who have managed so far in mainstream and do not see themselves as disabled are unwilling to go down this road. Some areas have integrated sports facilities in which everyone can take part at their own level; otherwise, young people should be encouraged to find another activity that is less physically challenging or competitive but will still help keep them fit.

It is also important to encourage young people to move towards independence. How far this can go will of course depend on the severity of their hemiplegia and whether they have associated problems such as learning difficulties, epilepsy or a visual impairment. Some may have complex support needs that mean they need a placement in a specialized residential school (see Chapter 8 for more about this) and possibly residential care as adults. But the majority of young people with hemiplegia should be able to do what their classmates are doing, with support as necessary – going on school trips, camping with Scouts or Guides and eventually with friends, learning to travel on public transport to school and other activities, and going shopping and to the cinema. Allow them to grow up – the fact that you have to help your daughter with her hair and nail polish does not mean she cannot go into town with her friends once it's done.

Sisters and brothers

Reading the parents' survey forms, I was particularly struck with the answers to one question: how their child's hemiplegia had affected any other children in the family. Some comments were very positive:

> Her big brother of seven years is very supportive. Also because he treats her like an equal, she (aged four) is more determined to do what he is doing.

> My younger brother is supportive and is always searching new potential treatments for me . . . My dad is amazing too – anything that can be done for me – he's done . . . It's definitely made my family stronger! (Adult with hemiplegia)

> They are very tolerant of others. They are educators of their peers and very often defend other children against bullying/comments.

Many more, however, talked about negative effects. It is natural that the child with hemiplegia will always be 'the special one' to parents, and will always need more care and attention than other children in the family. Brothers and sisters get less of their parents' attention, and are forced to fit in with the child's needs. The answers below are typical of many:

> *Numerous hospital appointments where the professionals always ignore M's sister or she is left with friends while we go to appointments. Physiotherapy at home takes time. Holidays are arranged around M's Botox injections.*

> *As I am a lone parent my younger daughter is often left to amuse herself and has to wait until I am free.*

> *I think that my daughter is sometimes jealous of the extra attention her brother receives and feels that I am stricter with her than with him.*

Another mother pointed out to me how parents need to realize how different a child's view of life can be. She would try to leave her elder son at his friend's house while she took his younger brother to therapy appointments, believing that he would find playing with his friend much more enjoyable than hanging around the hospital. But when he was older, he told her that he had felt his brother was going off with her to have fun, while he was left behind.

Nor is it just a question of less attention. Siblings may be expected to help with exercises and therapeutic play, or to remind their brother or sister about using their weak hand, or later on in childhood to take him or her to school or to babysit. They become, in other words, assistant carers.

A lot of this is of course true of all big brothers and sisters, but usually as the younger child grows up he or she becomes an equal companion. Indeed, it may be the child with hemiplegia who is the older one, and a younger brother or sister overtaking him or her physically or academically. In either case siblings have to deal with other children teasing or bullying their brother or sister, or the brother or sister's own difficult behaviour. Family outings are affected, or they may miss out on activities and friendships of their own.

> *We now avoid some children's play places/parks because he gets upset when other children push his little brother or stare.*

> *Her brother and sister are very curtailed in what they are able to do and also don't always want to have friends back home if L is being difficult.*

> *My disability has had a significant effect upon my brothers as I have often needed more attention. My stress and anxiety levels have tended to have a knock-on effect upon everybody in the household. (Adult with hemiplegia)*

It may seem obvious that families, while trying to do their best for their disabled child, should not neglect his or her siblings, but HemiHelp members' experience shows that this can be a very difficult thing to balance out, and something that parents need to be very aware of. HemiHelp has an information sheet, *Brothers and Sisters*, with suggestions on minimizing family tension, and there are several organizations that support siblings and help them feel less alone. Details can be found at the end of this chapter.

Family and friends

> *Because J's hemiplegia is quite mild, friends and family prefer to act as though he is fine (plus we are not good at asking for help).*

The survey showed that many families felt they lacked support from the very people they might most expect it from – their own families. This is often a result of people moving to another area and having no family members nearby, so grandparents may not see their grandchild very often and not fully understand how hemiplegia affects him or her. It can be easy to jump to the conclusion that bad behaviour is the result of bad parenting, for example, or that parents are just mollycoddling their child. On the other hand, family members and friends might want to help but be unsure how to do it. HemiHelp has a *Family and Friends* information sheet with suggestions on how parents can be helped and supported, and Contact a Family has a booklet for grandparents – both can be downloaded for free.

Talking to your child about hemiplegia
Some survey answers mentioned children, both those with hemiplegia and their brothers and sisters, wanting to know more about the condition and why it affected the one and not the other(s). Children, like their parents, need to be able to make sense of things, and I had the feeling that the families that were the most positive about their experience were those that had been open about it.

Of course, like other tricky subjects (sex education being the most obvious), the talking needs to be at the child's level. Apart from having their own questions answered, they need to have something to tell other children when asked, 'Why don't you use your right hand?' or 'What's that on your leg?' When my son was quite small he would happily say, 'My hand doesn't work very well. It's something I was born with.' and his playmates would be satisfied. Parents were sometimes more difficult – I remember the look of horror on the face of the mother of one of my son's friends when I told her that hemiplegia was caused by damage to the brain. Later, if something is not going well at school, for example if they find reading or maths more difficult than most of their classmates, learning that this, too, is part of hemiplegia can make it easier to accept, as long as they do not then think that they need not make an effort.

The process of learning about how hemiplegia affects a given child can continue into adulthood, although, with more early intervention, associated difficulties may be noticed earlier now than they were even quite recently. My son is now in his twenties, and it was only a few years ago that I realized that certain aspects of his behaviour could be described as being on the mild end of the autistic spectrum – not a concept that was around when he was a child even if we had noticed it. And he himself has started talking (and joking) about his obsessiveness and dislike of changes to routine. But adult life is another story, and another chapter.

Useful resources

Equipment, family activities, etc.

Radar (www.radar.org.uk) is the UK's largest disability campaigning organization. Their publications include *Doing Money Differently*, *Get Motoring*, and a guide to the National Key Scheme, which allows people with disabilities to use over 8000 locked toilets across the UK. (You can also order a key from the site.)

The Disabled Living Foundation (DLF) (www.dlf.org.uk) has a wide range of leaflets about practical solutions to everyday challenges, including choosing play and other equipment for children. It also runs disabled living centres around the country (go to www.assist-uk.org/centres for details) where equipment can be seen and tried out.

Remap (www.remap.org.uk) is the place to go if your child needs a special piece of equipment that is not available anywhere, or an adaptation to an existing piece. Remap works through a nationwide network of dedicated volunteers, who produce custom-made solutions free of charge for problems large and small.

Anything Left Handed (www.anythingleft-handed.co.uk) started as a shop in London but now operates as mail order only. It sells over 250 left-handed products, from scissors and non-smudge pens to computer mice, guitars and golf clubs. It also publishes information guides for parents and teachers (including a book, *The Left-handed Child*), and runs the Left-Handers Club, a free association of left-handers worldwide.

Get Kids Going! (www.getkidsgoing.com) is a charity that promotes sports for disabled children and young people by providing them with mobility equipment, mostly wheelchairs but also tricycles. It also supports their training, travel, etc.

Whizz-Kidz (www.whizz-kidz.org.uk) is another charity that provides mobility equipment, including tricycles.

Reach (www.reach.org.uk) was formed in 1978 by parents of children who were missing part of their arm or a hand, in order to lobby for the provision of artificial arms under the NHS. Since then it has grown to become a national organization providing support and advice for children with hand or arm deficiencies, and their parents. The website has a list of local groups (navigate to *About Reach*) and downloadable guides to driving, cycling and computers. Reach also has a hire scheme for one-handed recorders.

Wise Wheels (www.wisewheels.co.uk) supplies specialist cycles to children and adults with disabilities or mobility problems.

Disabled Living (www.disabledliving.co.uk) is based in Manchester, where it has an equipment centre with a wide range of products for use by people with disabilities. Among its other services is a holiday information pack with a list of companies and organizations offering accessible accommodation.

Special Needs Kids (www.special-needs-kids.co.uk) is an excellent information directory and shopping site listing products and services for children with special needs, including support groups, respite care, clothing, equipment, toys, leisure activities and days out, holidays and where to go for help and advice.

Child Disability Help (www.child-disability.co.uk) is a very informative website run by a parent of twins with cerebral palsy. Lots of links on practical issues – not only benefits, education, and so on, but also holidays and fun days out.

Fledglings (www.fledglings.org.uk) is a registered charity that helps parents and carers of a child with special needs of any kind to find simple, affordable solutions to practical problems. It offers a free product search service to locate toys, clothing, developmental aids and other items that may stimulate the child's development or give relief to the carer.

KIDS (www.kids.org.uk) aims to improve the lives of disabled children and their families. The charity is involved in providing services such as Portage and respite care, but is particularly associated with inclusive, often adventurous, play opportunities. It also runs projects to provide support for siblings and young carers.

Northern Ireland

The Cedar Foundation (www.cedar-foundation.org/index.cfm/section/top/page/YoungPeople; (028) 9066 6188; info@cedar-foundation.org) provides support, care, accommodation and training to enable disabled adults and children to participate in all aspects of community life. Services include short breaks for both families and children.

Parents Stories (www.parents-stories.co.uk) is a useful parent-run site for families with children with disabilities living in Northern Ireland. As well as stories there are links to useful organizations, activities, accessible days out, etc.

Respite/short breaks

Contact a Family (www.cafamily.org.uk/holidays.html) has information on your rights and a *Holidays, Play and Leisure* guide.

Special Needs Kids (www.special-needs-kids.co.uk/respitecare.htm; enquiries@special-needs-kids.co.uk) has a list of charities offering breaks.

Break (www.break-charity.org).

Kids Direct Short Breaks (www.directshortbreaks.org.uk)

Mencap (www.mencap.org.uk) provides respite care.

Short Breaks Network (www.shortbreaksnetwork.org.uk).

Sport: general

English Federation of Disability Sport (www.efds.co.uk) is the national federation for all those organizations that represent disabled people in sport in

England. It has a regional manager in each of the ten regions, who coordinates sports provision for people with a disability in that region.

The Federation of Disability Sport Wales (www.disability-sports-wales.org).

Scottish Disability Sport (www.scottishdisabilitysport.com).

Disability Sports NI (www.dsni.co.uk).

Cerebral Palsy Sport (www.cpsport.org): in England and Wales, promotes and seeks to increase sport and physical recreational opportunities for people with a disability and especially those who have cerebral palsy of any kind.

Sport: individual

Disability Football (www.disabilityfootball.co.uk) is a directory of disability football clubs.

Disability Rugby (rfu.com/AboutTheRFU/Inclusion/Disability.aspx): a growing number of Rugby Union teams have been creating disabled sections within mainstream clubs.

Riding for the Disabled Association (RDA) (www.rda.org.uk/groups.htm; 0845 658 1082; info@rda.org.uk): the web page provides a list of contact details by region (including Northern Ireland) with a list of links and telephone numbers to some of the county or local groups that provide horse riding opportunities for your child, from simply stroking a horse to having proper riding lessons.

Royal Yachting Association (RYA) (www.rya.org.uk; www.ryascotland.org.uk) runs Sailability 'to bring boating to people with disabilities'. It has regional organizers around the UK.

British Swimming (formerly the Amateur Swimming Association; www.britishswimming.org) runs Swim 21, an accreditation scheme for local clubs to encourage good practice and inclusion.

For other sports and more links, *Getting Active* is HemiHelp's information sheet on sports and other activities, downloadable from the website.

Arts

Sound Sense (www.soundsense.org): this community music organization now incorporates the National Music and Disability Information Service.

Living My Song (www.livingmysong.org.uk) is dedicated to exploring ways in which everyone can discover and express their own musical personality. Provides links to other useful websites.

Chickenshed (www.chickenshed.org.uk) is a groundbreaking theatre company for children and young people of all abilities and disabilities, which creates genuinely inclusive, high-quality and exciting performance. It started in 1974 in north London and now has 19 centres, mostly in England, but there is one in Scotland and two in Russia! It also runs workshops, courses and outreach projects. To see a list of Sheds follow the links *Outreach > Current Sheds*.

Drake Music (www.drakemusicproject.org) is a music and technology organization enabling disabled children and adults to play conventional musical instruments. Branches across the English regions and sister organizations in Scotland and Northern Ireland.

HemiHelp has an information sheet on *Music*, with suggestions about suitable instruments, etc.

Support for parents, siblings and other family members

Contact a Family (www.cafamily.org.uk/families/familyissues/): the family section has downloadable booklets for siblings, dads, grandparents, etc.

Family Lives (www.familylives.org.uk; parentsupport@familylives.org.uk) is a family support charity that works for, and with, parents, families, children and carers. Its services include a free 24-hour parent support line (Parentline, 0808 800 2222), a free online chat service, individual and couple support, parenting groups and workshops and information materials. It also runs a website for parents concerned about bullying (www.besomeonetotell.org.uk).

Young Carers (www.youngcarers.net): part of Princess Royal Trust for Carers.

Sibs (www.sibs.org.uk): for brothers and sisters of disabled children and adults.

KIDS (www.kids.org.uk): a charity that works with disabled children and their families.

Summary
- Bringing up your child may seem like a constant round of treatment and therapy, but family life will still go on.
- Unless your child's hemiplegia is very severe, he or she will develop in many ways at the same pace as most children – smiling, speaking, and developing skills with his or her unaffected side.
- Focus on your child's abilities rather than his or her disabilities.
- Live as 'normal' a life as possible with your child: go to the local parent and toddler groups, park and swimming pool. Later, learning to swim and ride a bicycle or tricycle will not only strengthen muscles, but allow him or her to keep up with friends.
- At home, involve your child in everyday activities such as cooking and tidying.
- Enjoy time together as a family, while making an allowance for your child's abilities and stamina. Look for disability discounts etc. at attractions.
- If your child's complex needs seriously affect your family life, regular short breaks/respite may benefit everyone. You also might want to consider a residential school placement.

- Encourage your child to find spare-time activities that will bring enjoyment and a sense of achievement. This will also boost his or her self confidence.

- As your child grows up, encourage him or her to become as independent as possible.

- Be aware of the effect that your child's hemiplegia and the extra attention he or she needs is having on other children in the family, and make sure you give special time to each child.

- Your family and friends may find it hard to understand your child's hemiplegia, and may, for example, blame emotional and behaviour difficulties on bad parenting. Explaining your child's hemiplegia to them (this handbook should help) may make it easier for them to offer you their help and support.

- You also need to be open about hemiplegia with your child and any other children in your family, keeping your explanations at the right level and adding more detail as they grow.

Chapter 8
Education*

Liz Barnes

Choosing a school for their child is one of the biggest decisions parents have to take, and if the child has a disability or additional support needs, it is even more important to get it right. Parents of children with hemiplegia need to be prepared to put a lot of effort into getting the best for their child.

> *Once the support was in place we were happy but it was a fight to get it and an ongoing fight to keep it in place!*
>
> *Make sure you ask all the questions you want to; there is no need to feel awed by professionals – it is your child and you are the only one with an emotional investment.*
>
> *You know your child best, and don't let the 'professionals' tell you they know what they are doing. Make sure they listen to you!*
>
> *You must keep in contact, don't always expect the school to, problems can easily be missed, especially the 'invisible' ones!*

In the last 30 or so years UK government policy has been to meet the needs of children with disabilities in the mainstream system, and most children with hemiplegia go to local schools. Special schools have been gradually phased out, although, as with many things, this depends to some extent on where the family lives – local authority policies vary around the country. The HemiHelp parents' survey showed 80% of children in mainstream schools, about 10% in a mainstream school with a special unit, and about

---

* By the time you read this some of the details of how children are supported in education may have changed. To find out more go to the Handbook Update page at www.hemihelp.org.uk

10% in a special school. But, by law, *all* early years settings, schools, colleges and universities must not treat a disabled child or young person 'less favourably' and must make 'reasonable adjustments' for disabled pupils and students.

The different parts of the UK have slightly different education systems, or sometimes use different names, for additional support arrangements, for example. The Scottish education system in particular works separately from those in the other UK countries. So this chapter will concentrate on general approaches to supporting children with hemiplegia, and provide directions to sources of more specific or local information and support.

What additional support needs might a child with hemiplegia have?
- Some children with hemiplegia have additional support needs because of *medical diagnoses*, such as epilepsy or a visual or hearing impairment.
- Most children will face clear *physical challenges*, such as
  - climbing stairs;
  - being jostled by other children;
  - collecting and eating school dinner;
  - taking off and putting on coats and shoes, and changing for physical education;
  - seating in the classroom – sitting straight, having enough space, etc.;
  - taking part in physical education and sports with their classmates;
  - doing practical work that needs two hands – also the school environment may be very right-handed, an extra challenge for children with right-sided hemiplegia;
  - tiredness.
- All these should be easy enough for teachers and assistants to understand and deal with. However, Professor Robert Goodman's research study showed that more than half of all children with hemiplegia also have *hidden difficulties* that can affect their learning. For example, a child may have more than usual difficulty with
  - literacy and/or numeracy;
  - staying with a task when there are distractions;
  - understanding or remembering more than one instruction at a time;
  - writing;
  - finding his or her way around school.
- In addition, some children will have *emotional or social problems* that can make school life more difficult: anxiety, irritability, difficulty in making and keeping friends.

Some of these issues may not yet be obvious when children begin their education, and may only appear as they move up the school and start to lag behind their classmates in one or other area of learning, for example, or in their emotional development. So it is not surprising that teachers at all levels sometimes find it difficult to get their heads round all the difficulties that may crop up, and parents may have to battle to get the extra help they believe their child needs.

Schools have to deal with children with a variety of additional needs, and can tend to approach their support issues by slotting them into categories: those with a physical impairment need support of one kind, those with academic delay need another, those with behavioural issues yet another. Children who do not fit easily into one category or the other, and that includes many children with hemiplegia, may fall between the cracks, and that is why it is important that parents and schools see themselves as partners in identifying and tackling additional support needs as they appear. The child's physiotherapist and occupational therapist can also provide advice. HemiHelp's *Guidelines for Teachers* pack is a useful tool that covers all the areas in which difficulties might arise and how best to address them, and there are links at the end of this chapter to other places to find useful information and advice.

> *Give them as much info as you can, we found the HemiHelp pack brilliant!*

> *The pack I got from HemiHelp has been a great help at school.*

Some children with hemiplegia have more complex support needs that may be difficult to meet in a mainstream setting. Depending on where the family lives, there may be a suitable special school in their area, but the trend towards inclusion has led to the closure of many of these, and moving out of mainstream may mean boarding at a school some distance away. This need not mean paying high fees – if the child has a Statement of Special Educational Needs, the local authority will pay if it can be shown that his or her needs cannot be met locally.

Early years
Parents may feel that they and their toddler are kept busy enough with visits to the child development centre/unit for various kinds of therapy, but a child with hemiplegia, just like any other child, is soon ready for playgroup, nursery or other early years setting. There they will benefit from meeting and playing with other children, and developing their language and social abilities, and self-care and motor skills. At this stage, aged two to three years, some children with hemiplegia will need more support than can be provided in a mainstream setting, but for many others this is the time when their difficulties will be least noticeable and when they can easily fit into a local nursery or playgroup. After all, many toddlers at this stage are clumsy or unsteady on their feet, or have the odd toilet accident.

> *Sending my boys to playschool was very emotional as they both were not walking. But, having said that, mixing with 'normal' children has done the boys' confidence a wonder of good. Within three weeks of attending playschool, their speech progressed and they both started walking!*

At the same time, with a high ratio of staff to children, nursery workers are well placed to notice any issues that should be tackled sooner rather than later – a visual or hearing impairment or visuospatial perception difficulty, for example. If extra help might be needed, parents can ask for a Statutory Assessment as soon as their child has reached his or her second birthday, and support at this stage will not only help the child's development but also make it easier to put continuing support in place as he or she moves up to school.

Throughout the UK children have a right to free pre-school education from the age of three years, usually for part of the day, and in Scotland and Wales this is the age at which they come into the education system. In Northern Ireland all pre-school settings (i.e. up to four years plus) come under health and social services rather than education, but the system for getting additional support works in the same way.

In England the early years structure changed in 2008, when the Early Years Foundation Stage (EYFS) was introduced, ending the distinction between learning and care for young children, and bringing together early learning and child care from birth to the child's fifth birthday into a single framework. This means that all early years providers, whether government-funded or not, and including childminders and crèches, have to go through an accreditation process and be registered with Ofsted. Pre-school children follow the Foundation Stage of the National Curriculum, and a detailed record is kept of every child's progress in all areas of their development. These include not just early language and counting, but also social skills, physical development and creativity.

Children with disabilities and/or special educational needs (or SEN) may also receive support at this stage through the Early Support Programme (see page 41). In theory, this attention to detail should mean that additional needs will be picked up earlier and that there will be more people trained to meet them, but it is too early to say whether this is the case.

Additional support

At the time of writing, getting extra help in an early years setting or at school in England, Wales or Northern Ireland is a three-stage process, which may lead to the child being given a Statement of Special Education Needs. In Scotland children are said to have Additional Support Needs (ASN) – the stages are slightly different and they may receive a Coordinated Support Plan (CSP). You can find a summary of the Scottish approach at the end of this section. Wherever the family lives, parents should be kept informed about their child's progress and consulted at each stage, and, if they are unhappy at any point, they should speak to the school or contact their local Parent Partnership Service. (See end of chapter for where to go for more detailed information.)

Stage 1 (Early Years Action and School Action)
Your child's school or setting may decide that the child needs extra or different help and they may have to use different ways of teaching, or provide the child with some support from an adult or access to technology.

Help such as this that comes from the school's own resources is referred to as 'Early Years Action' in early years settings and 'School Action' at school.

Stage 2 (Early Years Action Plus and School Action Plus)
If the support the child is receiving is not helping him or her progress enough, the teacher or the school's Special Educational Needs Coordinator (SENCo) should consult parents about additional support. This could be from a specialist teacher, an educational psychologist or a speech and language therapist, for example. Help such as this in early years settings is referred to as 'Early Years Action Plus', and when at school, 'School Action Plus'.

Stage 3 (Statutory Assessment)
For many children, support at stage 1 or 2 will be enough to help them make good progress, but some children will need more support than can be funded by the nursery or school. In this case, either the early years setting/school or the child's parents can ask the local authority to carry out a Statutory Assessment to help decide what more support he or she needs, and this support will be funded by the local authority through a Statement of Special Educational Needs. If the local authority agrees that the child does need this extra support, a Statement will be drawn up detailing this support. If it refuses, parents can appeal to their local Special Educational Needs Tribunal (SENDIST)

Getting a Statement
There is a fixed timetable for this process that differs from country to country; more information can be found in publications from both government departments and support organizations – for details see the end of this chapter.

Important things to remember when getting a statement

- All the child's needs – physical, emotional and educational – need to be included.
- The amount and type of support should be specific and detailed – for example, one-to-one support from an assistant 15 hours a week and a visit from a physiotherapist once a fortnight. Phrases such as 'physiotherapy as needed' are no good.
- If parents disagree with anything in the Statement, they can appeal to their local Special Educational Needs Tribunal (SENDIST). Parent Partnership Services can help with this, and some support organizations will provide not only information and advice but also someone to help parents present their case at a tribunal (see end of chapter).
- When the Statement is agreed parents have the right to choose their child's school. Some parents whose children were not making good process in a local mainstream school have persuaded their local authority to fund a place in a fee-paying special school.
- Even once the Statement is agreed, it can take time to put support in place.

- Statements are reviewed every year, so parents need to keep checking on their child's progress to see if anything needs changing, especially when they transfer from early years to primary and from primary to secondary education.
- Contact Parent Partnership and get the education authority on your side! Be tough and get someone to advocate for you. I was often frightened to speak out for R but when he got an advocate and I did it helped.
- Don't be worried about having a Statement – our experience so far that it only has a positive effect.

The Scottish approach to supporting children with additional needs
In most of the UK, children who need extra support in education are said to have 'special educational needs'. In Scotland, the Education (Additional Support for Learning) (Scotland) Act 2004, updated 2009, talks about 'additional support needs', a broader term that covers *anything* that makes it harder for the child to get to school and take part fully in the curriculum. And the local authority must make 'adequate and efficient' provision for young people who need extra help at school *for any reason*.

Additional support needs can include

- social or emotional difficulties,
- problems at home,
- being particularly gifted,
- a physical disability,
- moving house frequently,
- behavioural difficulties,
- bullying,
- a sensory impairment or communication problem,
- being a young carer or parent, or
- having English as a second language.

In general, the less formal levels of support are similar to the system in other parts of the UK – i.e. Early Years and School Action and Action Plus – and the type of help offered will be similar.

Some children will need a higher level of support. This is covered by the 'Co-ordinated Support Plan' (CSP). This is a formal document (equivalent to a Statement of Special Educational Needs in other parts of the UK). For this level of support, the child needs a formal assessment by the local authority.

The main thing that is different in Scotland is that in order to be awarded a CSP the child must have complex, multiple or significant support needs that require the support of more than one agency, e.g. social *and* health services *and* educational professionals. The wider Scottish definition of additional support needs means that the assessment takes into account anything in a child's social and family environment that might be affecting his or her learning. On the other hand it can make it more difficult for a child from a stable home and supportive family to get a CSP, whatever his or her physical and learning support needs.

If parents disagree with any decision relating to a CSP they can appeal to an Additional Support Needs tribunal (www.asntscotland.gov.uk).

Transition: Early Years to Primary

Transferring from nursery to primary school can be stressful for any child. For a child with hemiplegia it may be even more so. It is common for children with hemiplegia to be more than usually anxious, to like routine and dislike change. Some have visual perceptual difficulties that make finding their way around a new building difficult. And, of course, they may worry about being teased or bullied or not allowed enough time to change for physical education. Teachers, for their part, may still not have heard of hemiplegia and will not know what to expect. And, even if they can think of solutions to visible problems, they certainly will not be prepared for the 'hidden' ones.

Many children may already be in a nursery class attached to their primary school, which of course makes the transition easier. Or the child might be at a local nursery and moving up with friends. However, some children may have been at a specialized nursery in a different area, and parents need to think about where their needs will best be served. A school close to home will make it easier for the child to make and keep friendships.

It is important to plan ahead, to visit the school with the child in the term before transfer, to let him or her visit the classroom, to meet the SENCo and class teacher and discuss any concerns anyone may have. If the child has an individual support worker who is not transferring, the school needs to make sure that support is in place before term starts. The HemiHelp *Guidelines for Teachers* pack includes an *About Me* sheet, with space for a photograph, on which parents can give the school useful information about their child.

> *Visit VERY EARLY – any adaptations needed, e.g. ramps, even rails in toilets, take ages to be funded and the work done.*
>
> *Get the occupational therapist to walk round with the child to establish where there may be problems – they can implement change quickly.*
>
> *Give teachers and the Special Educational Needs team the HemiHelp pack. Say to teachers what you have found helpful, better to write it down, as a busy teacher won't always remember verbal instructions.*
>
> *Go in to teachers with a positive attitude. Talk about what your child can do, not what they can't. Encourage their independence as much as possible before they start*

school. Try to work as a team with the staff so that you continue with their work at home, be it using pencil grips, or if your child's target is to put a coat on by him or herself.

We found tiredness was one of the biggest issues and it can help to just explain to the teachers that a child with hemiplegia has to put in 100% more effort than an able bodied child just to move around.

Choosing a school

Most children with hemiplegia go to mainstream schools, and many do well, with or without extra support. Others with more complex difficulties may struggle in large classes, or be labelled lazy or disruptive. There is no easy answer – each school, like each child, is different, and you need to weigh up what you feel is most important and best for your child: academic success, care and support, being local to develop independence and make friendships easier. Some parents, in search of smaller classes, steel themselves to pay for private education, but have had mixed experiences. Private schools can

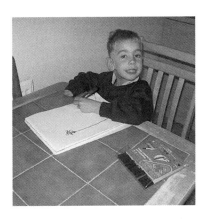

choose their pupils and some are not always interested in children who will need extra support and whose results might bring down their position in the league tables, whilst others may be very receptive. And private schools do not necessarily have more support resources than mainstream.

Our private school is very academic, but has been ten times better than our state school for pastoral care, to the extent they have even written the school timetable around B and how tired he will be after certain activities.

Unfortunately we chose a private school with little money for support. We wish we had chosen a mainstream school which would have been able to offer more support but we feel we cannot move him because emotionally this would be too traumatic. So he is in a school with people who love him and care for him but he doesn't receive a lot of help.

What to bear in mind when choosing a school

- Visit several schools, including one with a special unit.
- What is the building like – are there a lot of stairs or a complicated layout that might cause difficulties for your child? Ask the OT to visit if possible.
- Do you have an older child at the school who may smooth the way?
- What is the atmosphere like in the classrooms and playground? Are the children busy, happy and calm?

- Are there other children with disabilities or additional needs in the school? Talk to their parents.
- Does it have a close link with the senior school – to ease later transition
- Talk to the head and SENCo, and give them a copy of HemiHelp's pack. Are they interested in your child? Do they listen to you and ask questions about him or her?
- Are there clearly defined routines, rules and expectations? What is the policy on bullying?
- Remember that you are the expert on your child.

I chose my son's primary school because a friend took me along to see a Christmas show and I realized that every child in the school had a part. And the HemiHelp parents' survey echoed my feeling that the best school is one where inclusion and diversity are not just words out of a government code of practice. These comments are typical of many.

> *Talk to the head and SENCo and trust your instinct. The best school is the one that will be able to include your child in the best possible way. Your child will learn better if they are happy.*

> *If parents feel listened to and supported it is a good indication. Personal experience from an older child with no disability but educational needs has taught me that the environment and feel of the school is more important than educational results.*

> *It is really difficult knowing which choice to make, but remember you know your child best, and if things go horribly wrong you can make changes. You are not stuck with the same school for ever.*

Special schools
The question of whether a special school would be better for your child is also a complex one. Some children with hemiplegia will already have gone to a nursery specializing in children with additional needs, others may be just beginning to show delay in their learning development. They may be able to continue in mainstream in a special group or unit, or once they have a Statement of Special Educational Needs parents can ask for a placement at a special school. Some children even divide their time between mainstream and special schools. If you do decide that mainstream education cannot meet your child's needs, you then need to think about what type of special school will be most suitable. This means considering what your child's core special educational need is. It may be a specific learning difficulty such as dyslexia, it may be an autistic spectrum disorder, a visual impairment or severe epilepsy. In many cases it will be a combination of factors, some of which may emerge during their primary school years, and in many cases children start off in mainstream and switch to a special school as their additional needs are identified.

We found C suffered from low self-esteem at mainstream but since going to special school this has improved as he is not 'bottom of the pile'.

Try and get into a school specializing in cerebral palsy. They will get a lot more help than in mainstream. All the physiotherapy, [occupational therapy] and speech therapy is on site as well as the clinic for splints, etc.

However, with the closure of many special schools, especially those for less severely impaired children, there may not always be a suitable school locally, and your child may have to travel some distance, or if necessary board at a residential school. (The local authority will have to pay for this if you show that they cannot meet the child's needs locally.) This is a difficult decision for parents to make and many feel guilty about 'sending their child away', but for some children it may be the best option.

My son's residential special school specializes in challenging behaviour, but has been happy to provide for the therapy side of his hemiplegia as well.

It was the hardest decision we have ever had to take, but residential school has been great for M and great for us as a family.

For information and advice about choosing a special school, your local authority is a good first stop. There are links at the end of this chapter to directories of special schools, and if your child's support needs are connected with an additional diagnosis e.g. epilepsy, Asperger syndrome or learning disability, the charities dedicated to these conditions will also be able to help.

Primary years

Although there will be fewer adults around than in pre-school, children in primary school do have their own class teacher and classroom as a stable centre of school life. And, although teasing, bullying and being ignored can happen to any child, with or without a disability, children at this age are generally accepting of difference, and this is a good time for forming friendships that may carry a child through to the more tricky secondary stage.

R has suffered the full range from being 'left out' and ignored to being made fun of and physical bullying throughout primary school. He has coped by making friends with a small group of boys in the year below him who match him physically in size (he is small) and who are themselves outcasts (considered 'geeks').

He has good friends, he's grown up with some of them, they're always looking out for him. Like if he's climbing anything, they'll be in the queue, and they'll almost stop the queue to give him time to do it.

Many schools encourage children to talk about themselves in class, for example by having a circle time, so that a child with hemiplegia might, for example, tell classmates why he or she has to wear a splint, and another child might talk about getting glasses. Parents can also build up relationships with teachers, remembering that with each new year it might be necessary to explain everything from scratch. If they have time, many parents have found it useful to volunteer at school.

> *Speak to other parents; join the [parent–teacher association].*

> *I volunteered to help hear the children read. I was accepted by staff and children because I was regularly part of lessons even if I ignored my son at school. This helped me to overcome the lack of a Statement for T.*

> *It has helped being the Special Needs Governor at the school.*

> *Make a list beforehand of everything that you think might help your child to have a successful school year, no matter how far-fetched it may seem. Go to your meeting armed with this list, ask for the universe and you might just get the moon. Also, make sure that you are aware of all of your child's strengths and weaknesses*

> *Don't assume all Special Needs support offered is the right thing to take up for your child – is a specialist maths group set at your child's lowest performance level? Is being separated out in any way counterproductive because of the impact on their pride?*

As children progress through primary school, additional support needs may emerge. Difficulties with literacy and numeracy are common in children with hemiplegia, as are visual spatial problems. They may struggle with self-organization, find remembering things difficult, be easily distracted. Depending on the school, effective support may be easily obtained, or parents may find themselves battling for recognition of their child's difficulties. HemiHelp has a comprehensive *Guidelines for Teachers* pack for early years and primary school staff that members and schools have found a useful resource.

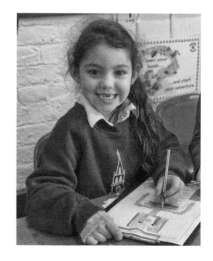

To give an idea of everyday support in the classroom, Martin, a year 6 teacher, describes how he and an assistant worked with a child with hemiplegia who was on School Action Plus:

> *P had additional resources to help him access the curriculum and be comfortable with sitting in class and manipulating smaller objects. He had his own chair, scissors, ruler and*

calculator, all designed to aid body position and fine motor skills. We did fine motor skills exercises with P on a regular basis, and also encouraged him to sit up straight, rest his arms on the table and push his chair in. We gave him large copies of paper, both for reading and writing, although sometimes he would use standard sizes. In art P needed particular support to slow down and take greater care and to recognize his difficulties with controlling the pencil or paint. P's organization was slow, and so we spent time packing his back pack, lunch box or physical education kit and generally chivvying him along. We would help with tying, fastening, zipping, and other children were exceptional in the way that they anticipated his needs and helped him without fuss. P would need encouragement to stay on task, focus, and not disappear into a parallel conversation about an unrelated topic. He needed particular attention after a disturbed night.

Key stage tests (SATs)

In those parts of the UK where pupils have formal key stage assessments or SATs (Standard Assessment Tests) at age 11 years, pupils who receive extra help in the classroom, whether or not they have a Statement of Special Educational Needs, may have additional support with their SATs. See the section on Examinations below.

Transition: primary to secondary

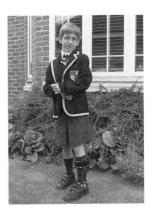

Choosing a secondary school can be tricky for anyone, and transition for children with additional needs requires even more thought and preparation. Secondary schools are generally much larger than primary schools: there are more buildings, more teachers and more students to cope with. Getting there may involve a bus or train journey with bags full of books, physical education gear, and so on. Otherwise the same questions apply as when choosing a primary school, although this time the child will be more involved in the decision. And, of course, it helps if he or she can go up with friends, or has a brother or sister at the same secondary school.

We looked at another school in the area, but he decided he wanted to go with his friends.

When she went to secondary school she didn't go with any friends, but she has an older brother and two older sisters in the same school, which helped. For instance someone was teasing her, calling her names, and one of her sisters sorted it out. And the boy who was doing it now supports her, which is nice.

Planning for transition should start at the child's year 5 review.

Children with Statements of Special Educational Needs go through the transition process separately, with the local authority offering a place at a school they consider suitable. But parents should beware. For example, the local authority may concentrate provision for pupils with special educational needs in a small number of schools. This is cheaper and easier for the local authority, and should mean that these schools are well resourced. For the child, it also means that he or she will not be the only student with a disability. But it can lead to a longer journey, overstretched facilities at these schools and a 'one size fits all' approach to support. Some children are provided with a free taxi service, but this creates problems with after-school activities and developing a social life with friends. Parents may also disagree with the local authority's choice for other reasons: for example, they may want a single-sex school for their daughter and be offered a place in a mixed school. Some parents may feel their child would be better off in a special school. As with any disagreement over a Statement of Special Educational Needs, it is possible to appeal to a tribunal.

More academically inclined children may want to take an entrance examination for a selective school, but it is important to check that the school will make the 'reasonable adjustments' needed to give the child a fair chance in the examination, for example rest breaks or the use of a keyboard.

Transition tips

- Start practising travel arrangements well in advance.
- A school visit from the physiotherapist or occupational therapist can be useful.
- Get into the habit of having books, physical education kit, etc. ready the evening before. It may be possible to have two sets of textbooks, one for home and one for school, to avoid too much carrying.
- Check where classes will be held: not all schools have lifts yet, so timetables need to be worked out to allow everything to be on the ground and possibly first floor.
- Pupils with hemiplegia should be allowed to
  1. leave class five minutes early (with homework already given) to avoid the stampede
  2. leave physical education lessons five minutes early to get changed
  3. have a card allowing them to leave the classroom to go to the toilet and to get lunch without queuing
  4. keep their things in a locker.

Secondary years

Learning

Secondary schools are less used to dealing with parents on a regular basis, but it is still crucial to be in touch with the school's SENCo and the child's class tutor, especially in the first year when he or she is settling down. Again, HemiHelp's *Guidance for Teachers* pack is a useful information tool. Students may turn out to need extra support as the demands of the secondary curriculum become clearer; some young people with hemiplegia who had little difficulty with learning at primary school level are less able to cope with the abstract concepts they meet at this stage. Some who managed without a Statement of Special Educational Needs earlier may need one, and an existing Statement may also need to be changed in line with changing needs. The mother of the boy whose support in year 6 was described by his teacher above continues his story into secondary school:

> *Anticipating that P would have a less easy time in secondary we tried to get a Statement when he was in Year 6. For a number of reasons this wasn't finalized straight away, so he went into Year 7 without a Statement, but still got lots of support, including a 'buddy' from Year 10 or 11 to look after him for the first week of term. At the end of the first two weeks I contacted the SENCo and she told me that the school had underestimated P's difficulties, so got his Statement sorted out and it was finally in place when he moved into Year 8. Since P has had his Statement I have noticed two main changes:*
>
> 1. *He now has a mentor, a teaching assistant who is in charge of all home/school liaison, so I now have a 'hotline' to the school and can immediately raise any concerns, from science homework to a forgotten sports shirt. His mentor can also contact me at any time if the school has any concerns.*
> 2. *Homework is now better tailored to his abilities, e.g. if the rest of the class have to do exercises 1–10, P may be asked to do 1–5. Teachers also give him enlarged worksheets to allow him to write answers more easily (his handwriting is not good). And if they forget, I send an email to his mentor and she sorts it out.*

Leaving childhood

The problem with secondary school, of course, is that it coincides with becoming a teenager, with all the upheavals that brings. It is a time when appearance becomes more important, differences more noticeable. It becomes more difficult for young people with hemiplegia to keep up with their classmates, especially in sport, and many of the people who completed the HemiHelp survey of adults with hemiplegia reported their secondary school years as the most difficult time of their lives:

> *Sometimes I found it hard to mix socially and people mimicked my limp which upset me. By the end of the day I was always extremely tired.*

> *My confidence level was greatly affected. Stairs and corridors were a nightmare due to my hemiplegia. I never wanted to take part in [physical education] and opted out in later years.*

> *Primary schooling was fine, possibly younger classmates didn't notice my hemiplegia, but I was bullied for most of my secondary schooling, socializing was a problem and physical lessons were hard.*

The survey did throw up some more positive memories of these years, although even these hint at a somewhat mixed experience:

I enjoyed most of my subjects, particularly languages, although I have always found maths and science difficult. I have always had full-time support and I still do in the 6th form – my mother had to fight quite hard for me to have this level of support.

It took me longer to complete assignments and I received extra time for timed assessments. My involvement in school life was active and extremely positive. I felt I fitted in well.

Subjects such as domestic science, physics and chemistry were challenging due to the manual skills required. But that also provided much needed humour!

My hemiplegia definitely created a lot of challenges and misunderstandings. However, I think these struggles gave me more self-awareness and perception.

Obviously a lot here depends on the individual student, his or her personality and the particular challenges he or she faces as a result of hemiplegia, be they physical, academic or emotional. And, of course, for many young people with hemiplegia, as for any teenager, studying loses out to computer games, television and going out with friends. At this stage parents may feel themselves struggling in two directions: fighting for proper support so that their son or daughter can do themselves justice on the one hand, while struggling to make her or him take schoolwork seriously on the other.

But certain things came up again and again in the survey, especially bullying, teasing and social difficulties and their effect on the student's confidence and self-esteem. Parents need to be aware that an increase in anxiety or irritability at home may reflect problems at school that they may need to tackle. It is also important to boost their son or daughter's confidence by helping them find things they can do and succeed at outside school (see Chapter 7).

Examinations

Students who are receiving additional support at school, whether or not they have a Statement of Special Educational Needs, may be given extra time for coursework and also certain 'special arrangements' for examinations. These have to be agreed with the examination authorities through the SENCo but may include any or all of the following:

- extra time,
- supervised rest breaks,
- a special seating arrangement or larger desk,
- use of a keyboard, and
- a reader or scribe.

Many students with hemiplegia are also not good at time planning, and this too can affect results:

When we tried one test without someone time planning the paper for him he failed it and the same test with time planning he passed with a good grade.

Transition to post-16 education

This should start with a review meeting in year 9 to discuss a transition plan, and may involve not only the family and school, but if necessary also local health and social services. Careers advice is also available throught the Directgov Young People website at Direct.gov.uk/en/YoungPeople/index.htm. The student may decide to leave school at age 16 (although there plans to raise the school-leaving age in England, Wales and Northern Ireland to age 18 by 2013), but if he or she stays in education there is the option either to stay at school or to move to a sixth-form college or a further education or specialist college:

- A **school sixth form** may be a good option for students who are uneasy about change, although schools may not offer a very broad range of subjects or qualifications.

- **Colleges** offer a wider choice of subjects and courses, and also give students a chance to reinvent themselves and make new friends in a new, more adult, environment – this can be especially good for young people who have had a difficult time at secondary school.

- Some young people with hemiplegia may find that a **specialist college**, possibly residential, best meets their needs. Bear in mind that if a student leaves school at 16 and goes to college, they get three years' funding, but will not then be able to be funded for another full-time three-year college course at 19 years. If, however, they stay at school until 19, they can get three years' funding at college. See the links at the end of the chapter for information on how to choose a suitable specialist college.

In all of these settings students are entitled to the support they need to put them on a level footing with other students. If they stay at school, Statements of Special Educational Needs or other support arrangements stay in place, but students wishing to go to a college will need to arrange support directly with the college. Young people and parents should visit a number of colleges well in advance and talk to the SENCo or learning support team to find out about attitudes to disability and support offered. College staff can then liaise with the school SENCo about the student's possible needs, and parents may also be asked to provide confirmation of their son or daughter's disability from a medical professional. The Directgov website mentioned above will also direct you to information on funding for specialist colleges.

At this stage the young person, wanting to be more independent, may not want to accept extra support, but parents may still find it helps to keep in touch with the college SENCo or learning support team, and the HemiHelp pack is still useful. As before, students should have special arrangements for exams and timed coursework.

Sixteen- to 18-year-olds in Scotland, Wales or Northern Ireland who stay in education may be eligible for Education Maintenance Allowance (EMA), a grant of up to £30 a week, if their family income is low. In England, the EMA scheme has been closed, but students between 16 and 19 years old in full-time education or training who are considered 'most in need' (this may include having a disability) may receive a bursary of up to £1200 a year. For more information and to apply for either of these go to www.direct.gov.uk/en/EducationAndLearning/14To19/MoneyToLearn/16to19bursary/index.htm.

Higher education

If university is something you are considering, don't discount it because of your hemiplegia – I firmly believe that no mountain is insurmountable.

Going to university is a fun and exciting time – as well as slightly daunting as it emphasizes the transition of responsibility between you and your parents. It can be tricky to deal with so remember not to give yourself a hard time.

In 2007–2008 only about 7% of UK students in the first year of their university course were known to have a disability, and out of these by far the largest group (40%) had dyslexia, with only 4% (just over 2000 students) known to have mobility difficulties. Ten years earlier fewer than 4% of students had a disability, so this is real progress, but numbers are still small, which may explain why support provision is patchy.

Leeds University, where I am lucky enough to go, has what must be one of the best disability services out there. Not only are they friendly and approachable (as the whole uni seems to be towards physically disabled people) but the service given in regards to exam provisions, note takers . . . anything you can think of really, is excellent. And because I'm disabled I've got guaranteed university accommodation for the duration of my stay too!

Essentially they haven't got a clue how to deal with me being disabled as I am the only one at the university (or who has ever been at the university!) with a physical disability of any kind, and the first to do my course.

Part of the problem is that, unlike teachers in schools and colleges, university staff do not need to have teacher training and may never have had to think about things such as disability and inclusion. I was shocked by the attitude of my son's head of department at art college, for example. She accepted him on the basis of his portfolio of work, but later told me that if she had known about his support needs she would never have given him a place. I more than once had to remind her about the Disability Discrimination Act and her duty not to treat him 'less favourably' than other students: in other words to provide the support that would enable him to show his abilities. And the quotes above, from the HemiHelp survey of its adult members, show that he is not the only student with hemiplegia to have met with a complete lack of understanding. But other students have had a much easier time – you just need to find the right place for you.

Choosing a university

At UK universities, courses for the same subject can be very different from one another, so the first thing is to look for the courses that you think will suit you, and then look at those universities' websites. All universities should have a written policy statement on students with disabilities, setting out what facilities they have, what their attitude is and what they are prepared to do. Go to open days, contacting the disability team in advance so that they can show you around. You can then ask questions and get a feel for the place and its attitudes to your disability. Find out, for example, whether you can live in halls for all three years if you decide you would like to, and whether you can record lectures on a Dictaphone.

> *I went with my parents to open days at all six universities I'd put on my UCAS [Universities and Colleges Admissions Service] form, but it was only at Essex that they showed me not just the lecture buildings and halls but the bar and shop as well. Everywhere else they looked shocked when I asked. That wasn't the only reason I chose to go there but it did help!*

> *Exeter's Disability Resources Centre was a big factor in choosing them. Before I started, they contacted me to arrange an interview about the sort of help I would need. I was honestly amazed at the level of help they provide, almost too much in some cases.*

> *For me the most important considerations concerned the location of my college (halls of residence) in relation to my departments at Durham, as I cannot walk terribly far. The university were understanding and I was given a place in my college of choice, which was also very centrally located to the city. I was (exceptionally) given a parking permit in my final term of first year, and throughout the two subsequent years.*

Going to university can mean leaving home and being independent for the first time. For young people with hemiplegia this is a bigger step than for most, and what is a challenge for some is an opportunity for others.

> *It was difficult living full time in campus accommodation, and in the end I had to move back home. Now I commute on a daily basis.*

> *As a teenager I decided I wanted to become an occupational therapist. This ambition gave me the motivation needed to work for the academic qualifications I required and I went to Southampton University where I had a great time. It proved I could live independently and now I cannot think of anything that I have not found a way to manage.*

> *The onus is usually on the student to ask for what they need: if the services don't know what you need, they can't help you. Hopefully an assessment at the beginning of your course should help to ascertain your needs, but I have found that I've realized I have slightly different needs as the years have progressed, and if this is the case it is important to keep the services informed.*

Funding for support at university
Unlike further education colleges, universities have no funding for special needs support; students have to access it themselves in the form of the Disabled Students' Allowance (DSA; see end of chapter for how to apply for this). There is a box about disability on both the Universities and Colleges Admissions Service (UCAS) form and the student loan application form, and if you tick it you should get a letter inviting you to claim DSA. The university disability unit will need to make a detailed assessment of your support needs. Once again, it is important to get all this under way as soon as possible, as it can take a long time to put support in place, especially since this is not something university departments are used to doing.

> Although I had got my DSA through well before the beginning of term they hadn't even started trying to find me a support assistant, and when I complained they suggested I share the person who was supporting a deaf student.

As well as teaching support, the DSA covers other useful items:

> I got a computer and printer with lots of software including a voice recognition package, an mp3 recorder to use in lectures, and I could claim for some books and materials and also ink cartridges and photocopying costs.

> For me the most helpful items were an ergonomic desk chair which I chose from a specialist chair shop, and a kind of small keypad (Dana by AlphaSmart), on which I typed up most of my lectures, as I type (one-handed) more quickly than I write by hand.

Distance learning
Some young people and adults with hemiplegia may prefer to continue their studies through distance learning, which gives the flexibility to work at your own pace from home. A wide range of courses and qualifications are available. The following are the main providers of this type of learning:

National Extension College (www.nec.ac.uk): GCSE (General Certificate of Secondary Education), A levels and a variety of vocational courses available. Study is paper-based.

Learndirect (www.learndirect.co.uk) was set up by the government-backed organization Ufi (University for Industry), and provides internet-based courses leading to everything from Certificates in Adult Literacy and Numeracy (maths and English), to National Vocational Qualifications (NVQs), degrees and masters degrees.

The **Open University** (www.open.ac.uk) is the UK university dedicated to distance learning. Students with disabilities may be entitled to financial support to help with course fees and Disabled Students Allowance to help cover study-related costs. Go to www.open.ac.uk/disability/index.php for info on services for disabled students.

Useful names and addresses

Government

UK (www.direct.gov.uk/en/EducationAndLearning); Helpline: 0800 328 5050: education and training for disabled people. An overview of the Special Educational Needs support system (except Scotland – see below). Click on *Learning and your rights: more information* to download official documents including the 2010 Equality Act and the Special Educational Needs Code of Practice, and also *SEN: A Guide for Parents and Carers,* and *Bridging the Gap: A Guide to the Disabled Students' Allowances*

Carers Direct (www.nhs.uk/CarersDirect/guide/practicalsupport/Pages/residential-special-schools.aspx) gives help with choosing a residential special school for your child.

Scotland (www.scotland.gov.uk/Topics/Education): search on Additional Support for Learning.

Wales (www.new.wales.gov.uk/topics/educationandskills): the Welsh Assembly website.

Northern Ireland (www.deni.gov.uk): follow the links *Home > Special educational needs > Guide for parents.*

Parents' Centre (www.parentscentre.gov.uk): the government's general parent information site, with lots of information and links. For specific information about special educational needs, follow the links *Education and learning > Special needs.* The site has links to information about publications, including the *SEN Guide,* in Arabic, Chinese, Gujarati, Punjabi, Turkish, Vietnamese, Bengali, Greek, Hindi, Somali and Urdu, with instructions on how to obtain them.

Directgov Young People *(*www.direct.gov.uk/en/YoungPeople/): the government-funded agency for young people aged 13–19 years, or up to 25 in the case of young people with a physical or learning disability. The site has a lot of information and advice on a range of issues (learning, work, housing, etc.), including a separate disability section and links to local services.

Where to apply for Disabled Students' Allowance (DSA)

England www.studentfinanceengland.co.uk

Scotland www.student-support-saas.gov.uk

Wales www.studentfinancewales.co.uk

Northern Ireland www.studentfinanceni.co.uk

Information and support for parents

Parent Partnership Services (www.parentpartnership.org.uk): local services that offer information, advice and support for parents/carers of children and young people with special educational needs, and can put parents in touch with other local organizations. Parent Partnership Services also have a role in making sure that parents' views are heard and understood, and that these views inform local policy and practice. Some parent partnerships are based in the voluntary sector, although most are based in their local authority or children's trust. However, all parent partnerships are at 'arm's length' from the local authority, and are able to provide impartial advice and support to parents. A link on the home page leads to information on services around the UK.

Advisory Centre for Education (ACE) (www.ace-ed.org.uk; helpline 0808 800 5793): a national charity that provides independent advice for parents/carers of children aged 5–16 years in state-funded education on a wide range of educational issues. Its site has downloadable booklets on such subjects as early years help, assessment and getting a Statement of Special Educational Needs.

BBC (www.bbc.co.uk/schools/parents/work/primary/sen)

Contact a Family (CAF) (www.cafamily.org.uk/education.html): the link to Contact a Family's education section, with information and comprehensive downloadable guides on special educational needs for each UK area.

Independent Panel for Special Education Advice (IPSEA) (www.ipsea.org.uk helpline 0800 0184016): a volunteer-based charity offering free and independent advice to parents of children with special educational needs in England and Wales. Its services include downloadable information and advice, support and representation in appeals to the Special Educational Needs and Disability Tribunal. It also offers disability discrimination advice and training in collaboration with the Equality and Human Rights Commission.

Network 81 (www.network81.org; helpline 0845 077 4055): this is a national network of parents working towards properly resourced inclusive education for children with special educational needs. Publish downloadable leaflets and a parents' guide to getting support, and also train volunteer 'befrienders' who can support parents at meetings and through the assessment procedures.

Special schools/colleges

Joseph Rowntree Foundation publishes *The Right Place: a parent's guide to choosing a residential special school,* downloadable at www.jrf.org.uk/sites/files/jrf/1859351506.pdf.

Special Needs UK (www.specialneedsuk.org) has an easily searchable online directory of special schools.

OAASIS (Office for Advice, Assistance, Support and Information on Special Needs) (www.oaasis.co.uk/Free_Publications_6/Finding_the_right_school): a resource for parents and professionals caring for children and young people with autism/Asperger syndrome and other learning disabilities.

COPE: Directory of Post-16 Residential Education and Training for Young People with Special Needs is available to buy from Amazon but is expensive; try your local library.

The **Association of National Specialist Colleges** (www.natspec.org.uk) has an online directory of colleges and how to apply to them

Henshaws College is a specialist college whose website has an informative guide to finding and funding special further education (www.henshaws.org.uk/public/funding-leaflet_new-images-no-crops.pdf).

Information on specialist colleges and courses can also be obtained by contacting relevant charities (see below).

Education Otherwise (www.education-otherwise.net; 0845 478 6345) provides information and advice on home schooling.

Scotland

Learning and Teaching Scotland (www.ltscotland.org.uk; 08700 100 297; enquiries@LTScotland.org.uk) is a government-funded organization for curriculum development in Scotland. Provides advice, support, resources and staff development to the education community. Includes *Parentzone* (www.ltscotland. org.uk/parentzone) – information for parents on all aspects of education, including additional support for learning (ASL).

Edinburgh Grid for Learning (http://egfl.net/): more information on ASL.

Enquire (www.enquire.org.uk; info@enquire.org.uk; helpline 0845 123 2303): Scottish advice service for additional support for learning. Publishes downloadable parents' guide to additional support for learning and various useful fact sheets.

Chip – Children in the Highlands Information Point (www.childreninthehighlands.com; 01463 711189; info@chipplus.org.uk): an information and support service set up for the Highlands region but useful for anyone in Scotland. Its publications include a parent information pack, a series of leaflets on how the additional support for learning system works and a transition guide for school leavers.

Wales

SNAP Cymru (www.snapcymru.org.uk; 0845 120 370; centraloffice@snapcymru.org): SNAP Cymru's independent Parent Partnership Service is free to families and offers accurate information, impartial advice and support to young people, parents and carers in Wales. It produces information not only in English and Welsh, but also in Arabic, Bengali, Chinese, French, Punjabi, Somali and Urdu.

Northern Ireland

Early Years (www.early-years.org; 028 9066 2825): a non-profit-making organization working since 1965 to promote high-quality services for children aged 0–12 years and their families, with an emphasis on inclusion and diversity. Provides information and training for parents, child-care providers, employers and local authorities, including a cross-border course on respecting difference. Based in Belfast with a number of regional offices and a network of local groups.

Cedar Foundation (NI) (www.cedar-foundation.org; 028 9066 6188; info@ cedar-foundation.org): organization providing support, care, accommodation and training services to enable disabled adults and children to participate in all aspects of community life. Offers excellent transition service.

Other disability organizations

Afasic (www.afasic.org.uk): an organization for people with speech and language impairment, but some information sheets are more widely relevant.

Being Dyslexic (www.beingdyslexic.co.uk): useful sections on additional support, for both parents/carers and teenagers/students.

British Dyslexia Association (www.bdadyslexia.org.uk/aboutdyslexia.html): information useful to parents whether or not their child has dyslexia.

Cerebra (www.cerebra.org.uk): follow the links *Parent support > Personal portfolios*. Cerebra offers a free service to help parents create a personal portfolio for their child, to provide information for schools, etc.

Dyspraxia Foundation (www.dyspraxiafoundation.org.uk): children with hemiplegia and dyspraxia have many similar difficulties at school.

Mencap (www.mencap.org.uk/statements): another good guide to getting a Statement of Special Educational Needs. Mencap also has a good families section with more education and other information.

Scope (www.scope.org.uk) runs a number of special schools, and has leaflets on a range of topics, including managing behaviour, fatigue, memory and visual perception difficulties.

Information and support for teachers
Parents and students may also find these sites useful.

Teachernet (www.teachernet.gov.uk): government site for teachers, with the latest information on special educational needs issues.

Joint Council for Qualifications (JCQ) (www.jcq.org.uk; 020 7638 4132; info@jcq.org.uk) has a downloadable booklet *Access Arrangements and Special Consideration*, with guidelines on examination arrangements.

Wales: **Welsh Joint Education Committee** (WJEC/CBAC) (www.wjec.co.uk; 029 2026 5000).

Northern Ireland: **Council for the Curriculum Examinations and Assessment** (CCEA) (www.ccea.org.uk; 02890 261200; info@ccea.org.uk).

Scotland: **Scottish Qualifications Agency** (www.sqa.org.uk): follow the links *Home > I am a. . . > Coordinator > Assessment Arrangements* (www.sqa.org.uk/sqa/14976.779.html)

Asperger Syndrome Foundation (www.aspergerfoundation.org.uk) has information sheets of relevance for teaching children with hemiplegia.

Dyspraxia Foundation (see above) has excellent interactive tables of issues that might arise at school and approaches to solving them: www.dyspraxiafoundation.org.uk/services/ed_classroom_guidelines.php (primary) www.dyspraxiafoundation.org.uk/services/ed_classroom_guidelines_09.php (secondary)

Equality Challenge Unit (www.ecu.ac.uk) promotes equality and diversity in higher education. Has downloadable guidance for academic staff.

National Association for Special Educational Needs (NASEN) (www.nasen.org.uk; 01827 311500; welcome@nasen.org.uk): with over 70 branches across the country, aims to promote the education, training, advancement and development of all those with additional support needs. Publications include journals and *The SEN Handbook for Trainee Teachers, NQTs and Teaching Assistants*.

SHIPS (Supporting Head Injured Pupils in School; www.shipsproject.org.uk; 0117 9673279) offers assessment of children after acquired brain injury (ABI), and training for educational professionals. Their site has advice sheets and other information, much of which is also applicable to teaching children with congenital hemiplegia.

Information and support for young people

Skill at Disability Alliance (www.disabilityalliance.org/skill.htm; helpline: 0800 328 5050; skill4disabledstudents@disabilityalliance.org) provides information and support for disabled students, their families and advisors.

Push (www.push.co.uk) is an irreverent online guide to universities. Search on 'disabilities' for articles and university profiles.

Yougo (www.ucas.ac.uk/yougo): UCAS (Universities and Colleges Admissions System) student information and social networking site.

Snowdon Award Scheme (www.snowdonawardscheme.org.uk/): awards grants to disabled students to help cover their extra costs. Available only to those who do not receive Disabled Students' Allowance.

Summary
- Most children with hemiplegia are in mainstream education.
- Your child will be ready for an early years setting at much the same age as typically developing children, although he or she may need extra support.
- If this is the case, early years staff are well placed to identify your child's needs and provide support that will then continue as he or she moves up to school.
- You should plan ahead and visit a range of schools before choosing one. A friendly and inclusive attitude to your child and his or her hemiplegia is as important as academic achievement.
- The physical challenges your child may face in school are predictable – stairs, physical education, school dinner – but in a more formal education environment it may also become clear that he or she needs support with the invisible difficulties that will affect learning (e.g. with literacy or numeracy).
- Some children will also have emotional and social difficulties that can affect their ability to make and keep friends.

- The level of support needed will depend on your child's difficulties, and may lead to a Statement of Special Education Needs, or in Scotland a Coordinated Support Plan (CSP).

- Some children with more complex needs may do best in a special school, day or residential.

- Planning for transition to secondary school should start in year 5, and again you need to look carefully at a range of schools to find the one that is best for your child.

- Secondary schools are larger and less friendly than primary schools. It helps if your child can move up with friends, or if an older sister or brother is at the same school.

- With a more challenging curriculum, your child's support needs may increase; keep in contact with the year tutor and SENCo to make sure these needs are being met.

- Adolescence is a tricky time for any young person, let alone for one with a disability. Self esteem can easily falter. Your child will need all your encouragement and understanding as they go through this time.

- School students who are receiving additional support may be given extra time for coursework and 'special arrangements' for examinations, e.g. extra time, use of a keyboard or a scribe

- At 16, young people with hemiplegia wanting to continue in education may choose to remain in school or transfer to a college. In either case they are still entitled to extra support. Some young people may find a specialist college, possibly residential, best meets their needs.

- Young adults aiming for higher education need to consider not only the courses offered by a given university, but also the facilities offered to disabled students and the general attitude to their hemiplegia.

- For those who find going to university daunting, there is the option of gaining qualifications through distance learning.

Chapter 9
Adult life

Liz Barnes

When, in 1990, the idea arose of a charity to support families living with hemiplegia, its aims included supporting young people with hemiplegia into adult life. However, its founding members all had young children, and naturally could not see so far into the future. Also, I think we all imagined that, with treatment and our increasing understanding of the condition, our sons and daughters would 'outgrow', or at least come to terms with, their difficulties and lead independent adult lives without the need for any further support. So the early trustees of HemiHelp decided to concentrate their efforts on providing information and support to parents with young children like their own, and those up to the age of 18 years.

But of course children with hemiplegia grow into adults with hemiplegia. And they find out that not only do their difficulties not go away, but also the support that they had as children may no longer be as easily available. So in 2003 HemiHelp decided to include them in its services, and set up a new category of adult membership (aged over 16 years). Since then it has been developing services for adult members, including a range of information sheets and 'Forward Thinking', a service to help young adults make the transition from education to independent adult life.

In 2008, as well as our parents' survey, we designed a survey for our adult members, and 169 of them completed it. A few of them are deep into middle age, but most are under 30. Their experience is reflected in this chapter, and you can also find out more about a few of our members who have written about themselves and their lives.

Work

My confidence has increased as time has gone on. I have found that people in the workplace have been less threatening towards me and my hemiplegia than the people were at school.

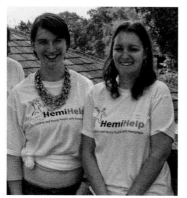

An important part of transition to adult life has always been leaving education and entering the workplace. Of the sample, the largest group, nearly half, were in work, one-third were still in education, and the rest, over 20%, were unemployed. The survey showed that people with hemiplegia do a wide variety of jobs: those mentioned include shop assistant, civil servant, barrister, occupational therapist, IT systems engineer, commis chef, bank cashier, teacher, public relations officer, petrol station attendant, theatre technician and receptionist.

Some HemiHelp members have found work without much difficulty and are happy in their jobs; others, especially those with more complex 'hidden' difficulties, have had a less easy time. The number of people without work is much higher than the national average, and while we do not know how typical the people were who took part in the survey, other studies have shown that unemployment is higher among disabled people than in the general population.

Many people, including employers, still believe that a national register of disabled people exists, alongside a quota system whereby companies must employ a certain number of disabled people. These disappeared in 1995 with the passing of the Disability Discrimination Act, which states that employers may not discriminate against people on grounds of disability – full stop. And the 2010 Equality Act further reinforced this 'equality duty'. There are a number of schemes run by both government agencies and voluntary organizations to support adults with more severe disabilities, especially learning disabilities, into and in work, although of course there are some people with hemiplegia whose severe and complex impairment mean they will never work in the outside world. However, the majority of people with hemiplegia will be competing for jobs with non-disabled candidates.

Davina, 24, teacher

Since I was very young I wanted to help others, so I enrolled onto a children's nursing course at Oxford Brookes University. I discussed at length with the tutors how my hand would affect me doing the course, and we all agreed that I could complete it, with adjustments if needed.

Then all of a sudden, after doing two years out of three, they said that I could not continue because of my right hand. It was true that I struggled with some procedures but I had always worked a way around them – it may have taken longer but I always managed to achieve my goal. It completely destroyed me and I lost all my confidence.

At my parents' suggestion I spent a few months travelling in Australia. I didn't particularly enjoy my trip, but I realize now that it forced me to get over my nursing. I still had no idea what I wanted to do, but after coming home I got a job in a holiday resort in Turkey, where I taught sailing and looked after children, and I was slowly able to build up my confidence again. I was then offered work in a Russian boarding school for underprivileged children affected by war and terrorism. It was an incredible experience because as soon as I arrived I was asked to teach all the children English from the ages of 10 to 17. I had never taught English before and could not speak a word of Russian, nor could the children or the teachers speak any English. I used every form of non-verbal communication to interact with everyone and I pretty fast learned how to speak Russian. I loved every second of it as all the children wanted to learn and were very appreciative of everyone and everything.

Back home, I tried to find a job working with children, but it was extremely difficult as I did not have many qualifications. I was concerned about undertaking another course as I did not want to fail again because of my right hand and being dyslexic. Then I found out about Montessori teaching. At my interview I told the tutors about my concerns, but they reassured me that I would be ok. I started the Montessori Diploma and finished in July 2009 with a distinction! After the uncertainty of the last few years I have managed to find a profession which I completely adore, and I am now working in a Montessori School in East London.

What I can say to other people is don't give up! Just keep on going and you will get there – if at first you don't succeed, try, try and try again!!!

HemiHelp members reported a mixed response to their hemiplegia from potential employers, but it was clear from their experiences that the more possible issues are discussed in advance, the less likely they are to arise on the job:

> *At work it has been people's misconceptions, judgments and 'unbelieving' that I have hemiplegia . . . only to find out that I do two weeks after they've hired me.*

> *I find that some employers handle the subject more sensitively than others, but I don't mind talking about it at all and I think it's necessary – employers need to establish that someone is capable of doing a job.*

At the same time many employers do not seem to know about their responsibilities – the Equality Act states that they must make 'reasonable adjustments' to working practices and the workplace itself so that disabled people are not at a disadvantage. This means everything from application forms to training to being able to use the canteen. This does not have to cost them anything – grants are available for adaptations to the workplace, specialized equipment such as a chair or keyboard, and so on, through the government '**Access to Work**' scheme (www.direct.gov.uk/en/DisabledPeople/Employmentsupport/WorkSchemesAndProgrammes/DG_4000347).

In practice, however, many employers simply do not understand what is required, even in the obvious area of access:

> *When I got my new job I was told they were moving into a new, more accessible, building, but when I went to see it the kitchen and meeting rooms were in the basement, one of the two ways down was by a spiral staircase and the other stairs were narrow and had a bend at the top. I needed to hold on to the rail, so I couldn't use either staircase if I was carrying papers or a cup. Fortunately they saw my point and hadn't yet signed the contract, so they didn't take it. But these were people actually trying to make their workplace accessible!*

But for many people with hemiplegia it is their 'hidden' difficulties that make getting and keeping work more difficult:

> *I had difficulties with finding and keeping a job due to inadequate social skills. I needed job coaching for several months but then I was able to manage a job without help.*

> *I was asked to leave the first couple of office jobs because of slowness/disorganization.*

> *I didn't realize how abrupt and rude I can come across when talking to others and having a short temper and taking things literally.*

One hopeful development is the government's **Positive about Disability** scheme: (www.direct.gov.uk/en/DisabledPeople/Employmentsupport/LookingForWork/DG_400 0314). This is a register of employers who welcome applications from disabled people and are positive about their abilities. For example, they promise to interview all disabled applicants who meet the minimum criteria for a job vacancy and to take action to promote disability awareness in all their employees. Registered employers, who include all government departments and many local authorities, display the scheme's 'Two Ticks' symbol on their application forms. The local Jobcentre Plus will have lists of local employers who are part of the scheme.

Someone with hemiplegia who is unemployed and looking for work can receive income-based Jobseekers' Allowance like anyone else, and Jobcentres have disability employment advisors who can offer help and support with getting into work. Anyone assessed as being unable to work may be able to claim Employment and Support Allowance (ESA). Depending on your circumstances, both of these may give access to housing and council tax benefits, as well as free prescriptions, sight tests and dental treatment.

Volunteering
Many young adults today, not just those with disabilities, have difficulty finding a job that suits them, and many find volunteering a good way of getting some useful

experience and improving their chances of employment. See links at the end of the chapter for organizations that can help.

Self-employment

Some people with hemiplegia have found it easier to set up a business or do other work from home. See the end of the chapter for useful links to help with a start up.

Go to (www.hemihelp.org.uk/hemiplegia/publications/leaflets/) to download *Getting into Work*, an information sheet that covers the area of employment in more detail.

Chris, office worker

I graduated from university not really knowing what I wanted or would be able to do. I'm still not sure where I want to end up, but for now I am in an office job and I hope this becomes a positive basis for me.

In my CV and in application forms for potential jobs, I have found it is better to explain how the condition has affected me personally and what help or consideration I would require from my employer. I feel this allows people to see not only how I cope and deal with the condition but also provides people with a more helpful explanation of hemiplegia than a medical dictionary could give.

Before I started my present job my managers met with me to chat about any alterations to my work pattern, desk, computer or access to the building. We agreed a plan to assist me where needed, with the proviso that I would let them know if I had any other problems. I now have my phone and computer set on the left side of my desk.

I have found that some of my colleagues do not have much positive experience of disability. People have asked me why I sometimes walk with a slight limp or with raised tone in my right side, but this does not affect or embarrass me any more.

If I were to offer any advice it would firstly be: do not be afraid to try anything, do something you are comfortable doing, and something you're passionate about. Doing something you don't want to purely because you feel hindered by hemiplegia isn't likely to be enjoyable.

Secondly: as far as you feel comfortable, be open about how hemiplegia affects you. Employers have a duty to help and assist you, and this may make your job prospects more accessible. With colleagues and friends, openness may help you get a healthy work /leisure balance – it could help your friends keep you included in activities if they are more aware of hemiplegia and you.

Benefits and financial help

Just as families with disabled children are, as a group, poorer than average, disabled adults are likely to earn less than non-disabled people with similar qualifications, while having higher living costs. There are, however, various benefits and concessions that they may be able to get. In many cases these are the same or similar to those available to families with children as listed in Chapter 5, so the descriptions below are brief. HemiHelp also has a downloadable information sheet, *Benefits and Financial Help for Adults*.

Disability Living Allowance (DLA)*

As for children, the main benefit available to adults with hemiplegia is the Disability Living Allowance. After the age of 16, it is the young person who has to apply, and if necessary appeal if they are at first refused or given a lower rate than they think their needs deserve. As an adult, it is no longer necessary to compare yourself with anyone; you simply need to have a long-term condition that affects your everyday activities.

Again, getting DLA may give you access to other help. In particular, getting the higher rate mobility component makes acquiring and running a car easier, whether or not you drive it yourself. See Chapter 5 and the section on Driving below for more information.

Young people aged 16-18 at school or college or on an approved job scheme who are getting DLA at any level may still be able to claim Employment and Support Allowance (ESA). However, the family may opt to continue to receive certain benefits such as Child Benefit and Child Tax Credit instead. Which is better depends on family income – in general the higher it is, the more it makes sense for the young person, rather than his or her parents, to claim benefits. Contact a Family (see links below) has a useful guide: *Money When your Child Reaches 16 Years of Age*.

Working Tax Credit

This is a benefit for people who are in work but with low earnings. Generally you need to be 25 or over to claim it, but if you are receiving DLA you can claim it from the age of 16, and if you get it at the highest rate you are entitled to an extra disability element. For details see www.hmrc.gov.uk/Taxcredits.

Other financial help

Some of this may depend on receiving Disability Living Allowance.

> **Grants for insulation and heating** Warm Front (England), Warm Deal (Scotland), Home Energy Efficiency Scheme (Wales) and Warm Homes Scheme (Northern Ireland) are a set of schemes for people on disability or income-related benefits.

---

* At the time of writing, The Government has proposed that DLA for those of working age (16-64 year olds) will be replaced by a new Personal Independence Payment from 2013. The Government plans also to stop paying DLA mobility component to adults in residential care from October 2012. To find out more go to the Handbook Update page at www.hemihelp.org.uk, or www.disabilityalliance.org/dlatest.htm

They provide grants for measures to make homes warmer, for example central heating.

VAT relief Disabled people can get VAT (value added tax) relief on home adaptations, specialized clothing, furniture, equipment, etc. related to their disability. You do not need to be receiving DLA or other disability benefits – you need only fill in a form saying that you have a disability, although HM Revenue & Customs (HMRC) have a right to inspect. For details see www.hmrc.gov.uk/vat/sectors/consumers/disabled.htm.

Disabled Facilities Grants (in Scotland, **Home Improvement Grants**) are means-tested awards available for making alterations to your home because of a disability. Contact your local authority. Scope (www.scope.org.uk) has a useful fact sheet.

Local authority benefits Although there is no longer a national disability register, your local authority may have a local register that gives the right to concessions for, for example, local leisure facilities, public transport or taxis, or a Blue Badge. Often 'disabled' is used to mean 'getting DLA', but each local authority has own rules.

Public transport A National Rail Pass gives a disabled person and one other adult one-third off ticket prices. Disabled people can travel for free on local buses throughout the UK.

Alex, occupational therapist

I have a right hemiplegia affecting both my arm and my leg but the lack of hand movement has had more impact on my life. As a child I attended mainstream schools – I was lucky that both at school and at home I was able to participate in all the usual activities of childhood, modified only where necessary, e.g. I played the glockenspiel at primary school with the recorder group. Looking back now as an adult I would say that the main impact my hemiplegia had on my life was not the physical difficulties as you might expect but the anxiety I suffered from, and still do, and the tiredness that came from the extra effort required to do everything. And I learned to dread shoe shopping with a passion!

It was as a teenager that I decided I wanted to become an occupational therapist. I don't think this was much influenced by my hemiplegia but I was inevitably more aware of the opportunity to find practical solutions to enable people to achieve independence. This ambition gave me the motivation needed to work for the academic qualifications I required and I went to Southampton University where I had a great time. It proved I could live independently and now I cannot think of anything that I have not found a way to manage.

From university I got a job in a large teaching hospital and later moved on to working in the community as a paediatric occupational therapist. This has given me the chance I always wanted to be able to use my unique position to help others achieve their potential. The main message that I want to pass on is that you can achieve your goals so long as you are prepared to persevere. I have learned to drive, live independently and travel around the world on holiday with friends.

Housing and social care

Most people with hemiplegia live in ordinary housing, with adaptations if necessary, and get by without help other than that given by family and friends, or paid for out of Disability Living Allowance.

Some, however, will need more financial and other support. Supported living may be an option; this allows people to live independently in the community but with support. This may, for example, mean employing a personal assistant for support with personal care and practical help in the home. While in the past such support was usually provided by social services, today disabled people are taking more control of their lives, through direct payments, individual budgets and self-directed care. Some people with complex support needs may need a residential placement.

The local council can tell you about its services and about supported or sheltered housing or residential care in your area. See the end of the chapter for other useful links.

Driving

Many people with hemiplegia can learn to drive, usually an automatic car with power steering and modifications to the controls as necessary (e.g. a steering ball, indicator lever extension, a pedal adaptation for those with right hemiplegia).

A visual impairment or a learning difficulty may be a barrier to becoming a driver, and anyone with epilepsy must be seizure-free for one year (with or without medication) to hold a licence. When applying for a provisional licence, epilepsy must be declared, along with hemiplegia and anything else that might affect the ability to drive. Go to www.direct.gov.uk/en/motoring and follow links to find out more about learning to drive and to download a medical form to send with your application.

You will then have to have an assessment to check whether you will be able to drive and what adaptations you will need. There is generally a charge for assessments, and prices vary from centre to centre. The Forum of Mobility Centres (www.mobility-centres.org.uk) has a network of centres around the UK and its website has all kinds of information and links for disabled drivers. Another useful organization is Mobilise (www.mobilise.info), which campaigns on behalf of disabled drivers and has an information service and a monthly magazine on all aspects of mobility.

If you are getting the Disability Living Allowance higher-rate mobility component

- you can learn to drive at age 16 years, and apply three months before that;
- you can lease or hire purchase a car through Motability (www.motability.co.uk), or, if you prefer, buy a car on a loan in the normal way and use your DLA to cover repayments (you do not have to drive the car yourself to access the scheme);
- you can apply for a Blue Badge for disabled parking, a street parking bay and road tax exemption (again, you do not have to drive yourself for this).

HemiHelp has an information sheet with more information about driving.

Katy, airport passenger service agent and HemiHelp trustee

I work at Stansted Airport for a handling agent called Servisair. We handle two different airlines from checking in and boarding to escorting unaccompanied minors. I have worked for Servisair for five years and the best thing about my job is the variety – when I walk in to work I never know what is going to happen – I love the 'buzz' of the atmosphere. The one downside is shift work – an early shift could see me starting at 3 am and a late shift at 7 pm.

Fortunately I can drive to work. When I started learning to drive I found it very challenging – but I got there eventually, after two years and four tests. I drive an automatic and I started with a steering ball and an extension on the left hand indicator but I now manage without them. I have driven many miles now, from Suffolk to Cornwall, and I love it.

I have quite a few hobbies – swimming, cycling, cooking, horse riding and also silk painting. I get a great sense of achievement from them all, which is really important if you have a disability because it helps build your confidence and self-esteem. But the thing I am proudest of is my Gold Duke of Edinburgh's Award. This award is designed so anyone can take part, so for example I went on an expedition with other people with special needs because with my hemiplegia and also hip problems I can't walk long distances.

Last year I went back into education. I am studying for a Foundation Degree in Playwork and Therapeutic Playwork. The first term was difficult because the University had failed to put into place the support I needed, but after that things went much better and after I complete it next year I hope to do a third year to get a BA and then a further degree to become a speech and language therapist.

My ultimate dream is to get married and have children in the future if I am lucky enough to find a special person who will love me for who I am and not see me with a disability.

Health and well-being

> *Basically the message is, be as proactive as you can. With hemiplegia, you exercise not to get fit, but to stay well.*

Unfortunately, there is little systematic health care aimed at adults with hemiplegia. Community services such as physiotherapy are designed to treat short-term situations – a fall, a broken limb – not chronic conditions, and those of our members who are receiving any regular treatment are usually having to pay for it. This does not mean that no treatment is available, and you should ask for a referral from your general practitioner if you have any specific aches and pains or, for example, think that an orthosis (splint) would help you walk. But it does mean that no one doctor or medical team will be keeping an eye on your condition, as happened when you were a child. At the same time, having hemiplegia puts more stress on the body and it is likely to age faster than average (see page 78 for more about this). It is therefore even more important for someone with hemiplegia to try to keep fit and healthy, and any medical intervention will be more effective if combined with regular exercise.

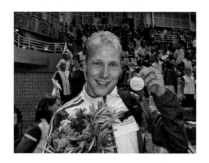

I took part in athletics and still hold the national record in long jump. I also did judo, which helped with my disability by learning about balance and how to fall. I focused on swimming as it got too much to do all sports, and I had more of a talent in swimming.
Sascha Kindred, Paralympic gold medallist

Not everyone is a natural athlete like Sascha and the other HemiHelp members who took part in (and brought home medals from) the 2008 Paralympic Games, but it is amazing how many different sports and activities our members are involved in, and mostly in mainstream settings. Cycling, swimming, and exercising at the gym, which exercise muscles without putting too much strain on joints, are particularly popular, but the list includes skiing, golf, bowls, rowing, horse riding, ballroom dancing, scuba diving, fencing, football, cricket, netball, aqua-aerobics, judo, karate, kayaking and canoeing. Activities such as yoga and Pilates develop flexibility and strengthen specific areas of the body, and at least two members of HemiHelp (only one of them female) swear by ballet as a way of developing balance and coordination. Obviously you should consult the instructors or coaches about what activities are suitable. The local authority may have a scheme giving disabled people concessionary rates for swimming pools, leisure centres and sports facilities.

Keeping fit is an important part of a general feeling of well-being, but it would be wrong to think that HemiHelp members are interested only in developing their abdominal muscles or their pirouettes. A few members with more severe hemiplegia and associated conditions reported difficulties with socializing, and some people mentioned only home-based non-social pursuits such as reading and computers, but most of the young adults who completed the survey seem to have pretty similar interests to others of the same age:

Swimming, computer games, socializing with friends.

Listening to music, going out to bars/clubs with friends, reading, swimming and going to the cinema.

Gym, out with friends, concerts, clubbing, cinema and shopping.

Chatting, giggling with my friends, thinking, philosophizing, learning . . . cooking and eating!

I do voluntary work, read – mostly work-related topics it seems! – and adore live music.

Friendships and relationships

This is an area that can present challenges for people with hemiplegia. Over 60% of the people who completed the HemiHelp survey felt that the condition affected their social life – it came second after education in the list of areas where they had encountered barriers. For many members it is other people's attitudes that limit choices, although on the positive side some report that in this respect things are better than when they were younger.

> *Older teens and adults are less focused on the disability and more focused on the person – disability can be a good filter for not so nice people*

Some people with hemiplegia have an Asperger-type difficulty in reading other people's reactions and feelings, a common enough aspect of hemiplegia that affects the ability to make and keep friends. Nevertheless, the typical answers above suggest that many members do have a social life and at least some friends. And another reason for taking part in sports and other group activities is that these provide a good opportunity to meet people with similar interests, who are more likely to become friends than just someone you met at work or in the pub.

As for personal relationships, there is nothing unusual in young adults feeling anxious about these, but having hemiplegia adds an extra layer of uncertainty, whether it is a question of appearance or lack of social confidence:

> *Doubts and fears are bound to come up surrounding sex. Talking your worries over with your partner is a great start – there are always ways around things – adaptation is the key.*

> *Until recently I didn't see myself as sexually attractive to men – so wouldn't even look at them as was convinced they'd think my arm and leg a turn-off!*

> *I have a boyfriend now but I do not have many other friends and do still have some social communication difficulties.*

> *Relationship difficulties – I am gay, and was extremely promiscuous at ages 18–21 – I was surprised people could find me attractive.*

There are, however, lots of people who have found their special person and realized that their hemiplegia need not be a turn-off. Melissa is one of them:

> *I have left-sided hemiplegia and am 25. When I first met Stu he asked me to play pool. I immediately panicked as I knew that he would see my bad arm. I said yes because I didn't want to be rude, but played the worst game of pool in my life! I tried to take the shots really quickly so he wouldn't see. We went out on a few dates after that and I never mentioned my disability. We were talking one night and Stuart said that he'd noticed my disability. It was actually a relief that he knew and I was pleasantly surprised that he wasn't bothered about it.*

That was ten years ago and we got married last August. He's brilliant. He puts my hair up for me, paints my nails and helps to iron my clothes. If we're out having a meal and I'm struggling to cut my food, he'll do it for me. I'm very stubborn and independent but he knows that if I need help, I'll ask. If I could give any advice for young people with hemiplegia on relationships, I would say be open and honest. You may feel that you want to hide it, but if someone sees that you're comfortable with who you are, that will overshadow your disability. I accept that there are things that I can't do, so I just concentrate on what I can do! My hemiplegia is part of me and has made me what I am today – I wouldn't want it any other way.

Parenthood

One of the subjects both parent and adult members of HemiHelp who took part in the surveys said they would like to read about was parenthood. There is no reason why people with hemiplegia should not become parents, and no greater risk of miscarriage or premature birth. And while hemiplegia can be passed on from parent to child, it happens very rarely. In general, you should follow the advice given to all potential parents about planning for a healthy baby:

Planning for a healthy baby

- If you have a partner, talk about any concerns and anxieties you may have and about sharing child-care roles and responsibilities.
- Get fit (even more important if you have a disability).
- Give up smoking and alcohol (fathers too – these can affect fertility in both men and women).
- Keep all the hospital appointments and discuss any possible issues with the midwives and doctors.
- Listen to your body – as the pregnancy goes on you will get tired and might need more help than usual.
- Think about any support and help you might need after the birth and get it organized in good time.

Given that HemiHelp has introduced services for adults with hemiplegia quite recently, most of our members in this category are in their teens and twenties, and not many are parents, but those who are a little older and have children are keen to recommend the experience. Here are three of them.

Jen, mother and HemiHelp helpliner

Just like all new mums, the thought of giving birth terrified me, but I gave birth naturally to all three boys. Hospital staff were very supportive. Although they didn't all have great knowledge of hemiplegia, when I explained my difficulties they did their utmost to help.

The worst part of pregnancy and just after the births (apart from intense tiredness and morning sickness) was not being able to support myself with my stomach muscles – getting out of bed etc. was more difficult for me because I don't have two arms to support me.

As a parent, my first major challenge was Andy making a bid for freedom when I changed his nappy. I soon discovered if I held him down with my right thigh he couldn't escape and he gave up trying when he knew I was bigger and stronger than he was. The other major challenge was car seats. They all need two hands to secure the baby, and were all too heavy for me to carry empty – never mind with baby enclosed! After much trial and error, I learned to use my teeth, my knees and occasionally my elbows! And with each subsequent child, the challenge began again and the knack returned!

Now Andy is a strapping 14-year-old blonde 5'4", Tom is 11, and although autistic is very lovable and funny, and Dan is eight, giving both his brothers a run for their money. Although they occasionally resent the fact that their mum has a disability, I believe it has led to them having far greater awareness and an independence most kids of their age can only dream of.

I'd advise anyone with hemiplegia who is considering parenthood to go for it. It's a scary experience for all new parents but my kids have enriched my life and brought so much joy. I wouldn't be without them.

Hugh, father and credit manager

The biggest challenge at first was not being able to help much. I was not able to pick up my child or to feed or change him. As our son has grown bigger and stronger over the years this ceased to matter and I am able to have a great relationship with him despite my hemiplegia. I am able to play with him and more importantly be with him and talk with him.

I can only speak from a man's point of view but, assuming the mother is prepared to take the major part in the early stages of child care, I would say don't hesitate to have a child. The rewards are far greater than any downsides.

Jane, mother

I'm 35 and have had right hemiplegia from birth. First of all, being a parent is fun whether you have hemiplegia or not. I have three lovely kids aged 15, 13 and 9. I don't think my hemiplegia has affected me being a parent at all, other than the normal limitations of hemiplegia. I did find whilst pregnant my balance was extra bad, but I managed OK with only a few falls, no harm done thankfully, and I had completely normal deliveries. I found my own ways of doing things when the kids were born, and made sure I was OK with any equipment bought (umbrella or flat-fold pushchairs I found easier, as they can be done one-handed and were lighter to put into a car). Anyone with a disability finds ways of doing everyday things that's easier for them – being a parent is no different. So if you are considering starting a family, go for it, there's no reason why you can't be just as good a Mum or Dad as anyone else.

Living with hemiplegia

It is clear that how easy or hard people have found adult life depends a lot on how hemiplegia affects them personally. With inclusion growing in education and the workplace, people with physical impairments are becoming more visible and more accepted as full members of society. Disabled characters are now regularly to be found in television soaps, and when a young woman born with an arm defect was given a job presenting a children's television programme there were only a few voices raised in protest. Of course, where a disability is not so visible, be it epilepsy or a learning, or especially a social, difficulty, acceptance is slower in coming.

But things are continuing to change. Dyslexia, for example, has not always been recognized: in the past if children had difficulties with reading they were just labelled 'thick' and sent off to do woodwork, or art if they were lucky. Now it is accepted that specific learning difficulties do not mean lack of intelligence. Schools and universities have strategies to help students, and, thanks to greater acceptance, not to mention spellcheckers and other software, it is less of an issue in the workplace. Over the last few years people have become much more aware of autistic spectrum disorders such as Asperger syndrome, and public understanding of these is also growing. We have to hope that in the future there will be more early intervention to identify and minimize the various difficulties that can come with hemiplegia, and that at the same time there will be greater acceptance of difference, so that the young children of today will face fewer barriers when they grow into adults.

But whatever barriers they have faced, or may still be facing, the young people who completed the survey are a pretty impressive bunch, and I would like to finish this chapter with some of the things they wrote about themselves and their life with hemiplegia.

If other people say horrible things, don't listen; it's them with the problem, not you!

My friends, family and I have learned that my hemiplegia needs a good level of patience and perseverance. I have been thankful that my friends and family have been educated by C the person rather than hemiplegia. Despite knowing the limitations hemiplegia places on me, they have been able to see how my life has hemiplegia rather than hemiplegia has my life.

I see myself as an able-bodied person, living an independent life to the full. I will ask for help if I need it, but most things I can do on my own (some things are easier to do with one hand anyway!).

Be yourself and try your hardest. Real friends will always help you. Don't ever doubt yourself just because other people may doubt your abilities.

Normally I don't think of myself as disabled but now and again something will smack me between the eyes. Usually the ignorance of others.

Some people may look at me when I wear my splint and think of me as 'disabled' – but disabled to me means dependency and that's not me. I know what I can do and what I can't – I can do lots of things independently . . . they just take longer!

I do consider myself to be disabled, I don't see why 'being disabled' is something to shy away from. I also think I identify with it as I believe in the social model of disability, which says that I'm disabled by the barriers within society (attitudes, etc.) not by my hemiplegia.

Sometimes it's hard having hemiplegia and it feels unfair, but you must keep faith that you're brilliant. You'll do just fine wherever you choose to go and whatever you choose to do. Having hemiplegia should not prevent you from leading a happy and satisfied life – and it'll probably make you quite wise!

More useful addresses

General

A Transition Guide for All Services (www.transitionnetwork.org.uk or www.everychildmatters.gov.uk): written for professionals but useful if you can wade through it.

Government site with information for disabled people (www.direct.gov.uk/en/DisabledPeople): information on services for all aspects of life, including employment, health, housing, leisure and transport.

Disability Alliance (www.disabilityalliance.org): aims to improve living standards of disabled people. Their annual *Disability Rights Handbook* contains everything you need to know about social security benefits and tax credits, as well as other areas such as social and residential care and a range of other issues relevant to disabled people and their families. It is for sale (at reduced cost to people receiving benefits), but much of the information is free to download from the website.

HemiHelp (www.hemihelp.org.uk): a variety of information sheets for adults with hemiplegia, 'Forward Thinking', a mentoring service to support young adults in their transition to work or higher education, a Facebook group (search for HemiHelp at www.facebook.com) and an over-16 message board thread at www.hemihelp.org.uk. You can also tweet @hemihelp.

Scope (www.scope.org.uk): a range of useful information for young adults, including *My Money, My Way*, a young person's guide to direct payments. It also provides a support service to help people into employment (www.scope.org.uk/ services/employment-service), although this is not available in all areas, as well as supported independent living and residential care services,

Work

Government site with information on work schemes and programmes (www.direct.gov.uk/en/DisabledPeople/Employmentsupport/WorkSchemes AndProgrammes)

Association of Disabled Professionals (www.adp.org.uk; info@adp.org.uk): provides advice, information and peer support on education, training and employment.

Disabled Entrepreneurs Network (www.disabled-entrepreneurs.net): provides networking opportunities and information services for self-employed disabled people through its regional groups. Publishes a *Resource Guide*, *Directory of Support* and *Quick Reference Guide* which is free to anyone with a disability.

Shell LiveWIRE (www.shell-livewire.org): another site offering information and advice on setting up in business.

Employment Opportunities (www.opportunities.org.uk): part of national employment charity Shaw Trust, dedicated to creating routes into employment for people with all types of disability

Sheffield Hallam University Access to Work guide (students.shu.ac.uk/services/ disability/docs/Access_to_work.pdf) A useful booklet about the Access to Work scheme.

Volunteering

Government site (www.direct.gov.uk/en/HomeAndCommunity/Gettinginvolvedinyourcommunity/ Volunteering/index.htm).

Community Service Volunteers (www.csv.org.uk).

YouthNet (www.youthnet.org): an online charity offering guidance and support to young people aged 16–24. Has a volunteering section (www.do-it.org).

Volunteering England (www.volunteering.org.uk).

Volunteer Development Scotland (www.vds.org.uk).

Volunteering Wales (www.volunteering-wales.net/index.html).

Volunteer Development Agency (Northern Ireland; www.volunteering-ni.org).

Benefits

Contact a Family (www.cafamily.org.uk/pdfs/Checklists.pdf): downloadable booklets on Employment and Support Allowance (ESA), transition, benefits, sex and relationships. Transition guidance covers the whole of the UK.

Benefits and Work (www.benefitsandwork.co.uk): an independent subscription site offering tips and tactics for applying for Disability Living Allowance, Employment and Support Allowance, etc.

Government information (www.direct.gov.uk/en/MoneyTaxAndBenefits/Benefits TaxCreditsAndOtherSupport/Disabledpeople/DG_10011925): go here to fill in or download a Disability Living Allowance form.

Department for Work and Pensions (www.dwp.gov.uk/publications/specialist-guides/decision-makers-guide/): click on Volume 10 to be sneaky and read the guide used by the decision makers when awarding Disability Living Allowance.

Turn2Us (www.turn2us.org.uk): another site to help you find out about benefits, grants and other financial help, including managing money. Has an easy-to-use benefits checker and a grants search section containing the details of hundreds of grant-giving charities (national, regional and local) that may be able to provide financial support and other services.

Disability Law Service (www.dls.org.uk ; advice line 020 7791 9800; advice@dls.org.uk) is a charity run by and for disabled people to provide advice and information on the law as regards disability, benefits, employment, etc. Their site has range of fact sheets and they also provide a casework service, and support at any level of the legal system.

Housing and social care

Housing Options (www.housingoptions.org.uk; 0845 4561497; enquiries@ housingoptions.org.uk) is a housing advisory service for people with learning disabilities.

In Control (www.in-control.org.uk) is a social enterprise that was set up to transform the current social care system into a system of self-directed support and individual budgets, giving disabled people as much control as possible of their lives. The website has fact sheets on how it works, and also on getting a job.

Independent Living Alternatives (www.ilanet.co.uk; 020 8906 9265) provides information on support services, employing personal assistants, advocacy and rights.

Independent Living Fund (www.ilf.org.uk) gives grants to people with severe disabilities, aged 16 and over, to buy services and equipment that enable them to maintain an independent lifestyle.

The National Centre for Independent Living (NCIL; www.ncil.org.uk; advice line 0845 026 4748) aims to promote independent living by providing support and information around Direct Payments and Individual Budgets. Resources include a directory of local support services and an employers' kit that helps employers and prospective employers with issues around employing staff on a direct payment or individual budget.

ITCH (www.itcanhelp.org.uk) is a network of volunteers who are able to offer free local computer assistance to disabled people. To contact your local volunteer, go to the site or telephone 0800 269545.

Independent Living (www.independentliving.co.uk) provides information about products and services to help with mobility and independence.

Totally Yours (www.totallyyours.co.uk) is a wide-ranging directory of product and service providers

Charities providing **adult residential care** services and information about residential care include the following:

Mencap (www.mencap.org.uk)

The National Autistic Society (www.autism.org.uk)

Leonard Cheshire Disability (www.lcdisability.org): for people with physical disabilities. Also runs a service users' independent organization called the Service User Networking Association (SUNA)

Health, leisure and well-being

The Bobath Centre, London (www.bobath.org.uk/adultpatients.php) treats mainly children with all types of cerebral palsy, including hemiplegia, but also runs a centre for adults with neurological disabilities. The centre is not part of the NHS, but NHS funding may be available on referral by a general practitioner or consultant.

Different Strokes (www.differentstrokes.co.uk): with branches around the UK, this organization is run by younger stroke survivors for younger stroke survivors, to encourage self-help and mutual support. Their site has downloadable information packs on services and benefits for adults. Their exercise classes will welcome all HemiHelp members.

See also **HemiHelp**'s information sheet *Staying Active*, on sport and active leisure opportunities.

Disability Arts (www.disabilityartsonline.org) is a relatively new art movement that reflects disabled people's perspective on the arts. Has a national directory of disability arts organizations, websites, etc.

RNIB leisure and culture information (www.rnib.org.uk/livingwithsightloss/leisureculture/Pages/leisure_culture. aspx): This is part of the RNIB (Royal National Institute of Blind People) website but has information useful for any disabled people on concessionary and free tickets, access, and so on for arts and music venues, especially in the London area.

Ableize (www.ableize.com) has a wide-ranging directory of UK disability resources. Find products and services, sports and holidays, and education, mobility, walking, living and bathing aids. The site is owned, run and maintained by disabled people.

Ouch! (www.bbc.co.uk/ouch) is a website from the BBC that reflects the lives and experiences of disabled people. It has articles, blogs, a very busy message board and an award-winning downloadable radio show – *The Ouch Podcast*.

DisabledGo (www.disabledgo.info) was set up by disabled people to remove barriers to mobility by providing accessibility guides to locations and venues across the UK and now in Europe too. Their fantastic site tells you everything you want to know about any given town or city, from loos to clubbing, and has a guide to university and college campuses – accommodation, bars, sports facilities, the lot!

Good Access Guide (www.goodaccessguide.co.uk) has a directory of services, from leisure and holidays to voluntary organizations in your area.

Enable Holidays (www.enableholidays.com) is a mainstream tour operator offering a specially selected range of overseas resorts and holiday accommodation to meet the needs of people with mobility impairments.

Parenthood

Disabled Parents Network (www.disabledparentsnetwork.org.uk) provides information, advice and peer support to disabled parents, their families and supporters. It also campaigns on a local and national level to improve services for disabled parents and provides training for social and health professionals.

Disability, Pregnancy and Parenthood International (DPPI) (www.dppi.org.uk) is the UK's national information charity on disability and parenthood and the publisher of the journal *Disability, Pregnancy & Parenthood International*. Their publications include *One Handed Parenting: a Practical Guide for New Parents*, available via their website or by calling 0800 018 4730, free to disabled parents and parents-to-be.

Mums With Disability (www.mumswithdisability.co.uk) is a social networking site with message board.

Summary

- In this chapter a number of HemiHelp members write about their experience of adult life

- As young people with hemiplegia grow up, they often discover that adult support services are less easy to access than children's ones were.

- Since 2003, HemiHelp has had a separate category of adult membership, with a range of information materials and a transition mentoring service.

- Disabled adults as a group are more likely to be out of work than the population as a whole; however, HemiHelp members are to be found in a wide range of employment.

- Under UK legislation, employers must not discriminate against people on grounds of disability, but many do not understand what this means.

- HemiHelp members have had a variety of responses to their condition from potential employers, but in general have found that being open about their hemiplegia from the start has helped avoid problems later.

- Someone with hemiplegia who is unemployed and looking for work can receive income-based Jobseekers' Allowance. Anyone assessed as being unable to work may be able to claim Employment and Support Allowance (ESA). Depending on your circumstances, both of these may give access to housing and council tax benefits, as well as free prescriptions, sight tests and dental treatment.

- The main benefit for adults with hemiplegia remains Disability Living Allowance (DLA), which young people need to claim for themselves from the age of 16. As with children, getting DLA can give access to further financial and other help.

- Most adults with hemiplegia live in ordinary housing, and pay for help out of their DLA if necessary. A few will need more financial and other support, which they will usually pay for through direct payments and personal budgets.

- Many people with hemiplegia can learn to drive, usually an automatic car with power steering and modifications to the controls as necessary. Before getting a provisional licence you need to have an assessment of your needs.

- People receiving DLA higher-rate mobility component can learn to drive at 16, lease a car through the Motability scheme and, with a Blue Badge, avoid road tax and parking charges (even if someone else drives the car).

- Having hemiplegia puts more stress on the body and it is likely to age faster than average. It is therefore even more important for someone with hemiplegia to try to keep fit and healthy.

- HemiHelp members are involved in a wide range of active pursuits, and some of them have won medals at the Paralympics (this is not obligatory).

- Some people with hemiplegia have difficulties with friendship, often through a lack of confidence (though other peoples' attitudes are also a factor), but many have good social lives and relationships.

- There is no reason why people with hemiplegia should not become parents, and no greater risk of miscarriage or premature birth. And while hemiplegia can be passed on from parent to child, it happens very rarely.

Chapter 10

The emotional impact of having a child with a disability

Claire Edwards

As parents of children with a disability, one aspect of our lives that is powerfully present but often appears to be ignored or diminished is that of the emotional impact. In this chapter I want to explore some of the issues related to this aspect. In doing so I will draw on my personal experience as a mother of a boy with Down syndrome and autistic features and my work with families for a parent-led voluntary organization in Scotland.

Becoming a parent

Becoming a parent is an incredible thing. Personally, I found the prospect of going into labour terrifying enough, let alone becoming responsible for another human being. What is clear, however, is that from the outset we are dealing with emotions – be it fear, excitement, anger, relief, delight or dread. Moreover, all of these, and many others you can no doubt think of, can be experienced at any time by the prospective parent – sometimes all within the space of ten minutes! Where there are two people involved, there is no guarantee that they will be feeling the same way at the same time. Actually, that is likely to be true pretty much from this point onwards (and usually prior to it too), but I will return to this aspect of parenthood later in the chapter.

Generally speaking, where the pregnancy is wanted then we can find ourselves attaching a range of attributes to our potential child and to ourselves as parents. Ambitions and aspirations, notions that surprise us, can take hold. This is a natural part of the process of adapting to our new role and new life and can occur whether we are becoming parents for the first time or are getting to be 'old hands'. Moreover, our ability to express and articulate these dreams and fears will vary, depending on so many other aspects of our life and our individual psychological make-up.

Our baby's arrival, therefore, can trigger a whole range of responses from us, related to these dreams and fears. If it is apparent at birth that our baby has difficulties, then we begin on a very particular journey – not having the baby we expected and quite possibly then not having the life we imagined in any shape or form we can recognize. Should it become apparent over time that our child is not reaching his or her milestones, then we have that particular additional adjustment to make. However it occurs, the experience will be accompanied by feelings and these can include loss, grief, anxiety and anger.

What do we feel about disability?
Sometimes these feelings can threaten to overwhelm us, and part of this stems from how we feel about our child. Generally speaking there is an intensity of feeling towards our children quite unlike any other, and this includes negative as well as positive feelings. This in itself can be profoundly challenging for us. Add potential disability into that picture and the emotional landscape becomes an increasingly complex one.

Parents of children with disabilities are no better prepared or equipped than other parents. Even if they already have direct experience of disability, being a parent is a whole different ball game. We are part of the society in which we live, and in the main that society has at best an ambivalent attitude towards disability.

As a society, our exposure to disability has been mixed and largely ill informed. While the move from confining disabled children and adults to institutions, to children living with their families and 'care in the community' can be seen as evidence of a progressive and enlightened society, we were woefully unprepared for it. Education and understanding was largely inadequate and sporadic in nature. Sadly, this continues to be the case today, in spite of the important efforts of the charitable and voluntary sector associated with disability and agencies within the statutory sector. We need to recognize this to understand the ambivalence I referred to earlier, and other attitudes such as anxiety, prejudice, fear and revulsion.

As parents we may have these attitudes ourselves – indeed few of us would claim to be free from prejudice and making judgements, even if we might not label our feelings in this way. How challenging then to find ourselves the parents of child with additional needs. Indeed this scenario can lead to many of us struggling at times to feel and be positive about our child, to send the message 'I love you as you are' when we may actually feel something quite different.

Given the context that most of us are operating in – living in a society that is ambivalent, with a relatively recent history of 'hiding away' those that did not fit perceptions of normality, is it any surprise that we might struggle with the circumstances of our life? What we feel can be challenging and distressing but it does not make us bad people. What matters is what we do with those feelings.

Acknowledgement of them by ourselves and those around us is an essential step in the process of making sense and coming to terms with the child that we have. This is perhaps easier to say than to do, not least because, while we can look at ourselves and reflect on our own feelings and attitudes, we also have to deal with, and have little control over, those expressed by others around us.

Our experiences are unique to us, but, without denying the individual nature of being human, we can identify some shared experiences and emotions that we have in common as parents of disabled children. Indeed the very language we use serves as a starting point. Many parents are uncomfortable with the term 'disability', particularly when their child is very young. Other terms such as 'difficulties',' special needs' or 'additional support needs' can feel more comfortable, perhaps more so when there is no confirmed diagnosis and the process of investigation has only just begun. I am using the word 'disability' with ease here because I also understand that the term refers to the way my child is perceived by the world around him. He undeniably has an impairment, but half the struggle is the disabling aspects of society: people's attitudes, the lack of compassion and apparent readiness to judge, and the battles that have to be fought along the way. Again, experiences will be different, but many parents report that they have to fight to get the right education for their child, short breaks, therapeutic treatments and social opportunities. What other explanation for this is there, other than a questioning of the child's right to be living as full a life as any other child?

This view may seem stark and uncompromising, but I state it because for many parents the lack of welcome for their child, or their perception of it, can haunt their sense of themselves as parents and impact on the way their family functions.

I also need to speak here of celebration, joy and delight. If a process of adjustment is made, preferably supported and encouraged by those around us, then many parents enjoy their child, marvel at his or her achievements and celebrate successes. But we will return to joy again later.

Being part of a community
None of us exist in isolation, although becoming a parent of a disabled child can feel pretty isolating at times. My emphasis on the society we live in is to acknowledge this but also then to comment on the smaller communities that most of us are a part of – our family and friends. One of the most helpful and, on reflection, powerful bits of advice I received early on was that others would take a lead from how I treated and responded to my child. The pressure was then on to display something positive to the world. I was in a position to do this as I received a great deal of support from some family and friends. As part of that process the weeping stopped (for a while), we had a party in the hospital to celebrate my son's arrival and, for the most part, those who came rose to the occasion.

I know, however, other parents who were not in a place to do that, as their child was ill or the trauma they had gone through was too great and immediate. Moreover, as I hope is clear here, it was possible for us because of the support we received – not everyone has that. Indeed the very people you need and expect to be there for you can, through fear, ignorance or maybe denial, turn from you. The saying 'in a crisis you find out who your friends are' can be oh so sadly true. Moreover, for many families the crises just keep on coming and one never, ever gets used to it . . . while for some of those around you compassion fatigue can set in.

'Getting with the system'

Becoming a parent of a disabled child requires us to engage with a host of professionals and services. Any parent has to get to grips with a range of systems and processes in meeting their parental responsibilities towards their child. Undeniably, though, we have to deal with more and are under greater scrutiny, be it in applying for Disability Living Allowance, being assessed for respite care, finding the appropriate educational placement, getting a Statement of Special Educational Needs for your child (England, Wales and Northern Ireland) or a Coordinated Support Plan (Scotland).

Two things in particular strike me about interactions between professionals and parents. Firstly, how often the emotional impact goes unacknowledged, and here I am also referring to the impact on the practitioner. Secondly, following this, how powerful it is when a practitioner does enquire and then acknowledge this impact. In addition, it can be profoundly helpful if this is done without any implication that if they were the parent of your child they would do a much better job than you are. Quite often we are feeling badly enough about our parenting skills as it is! This is not my personal experience talking here, but unfortunately a perception reported too often by parents I have spoken to over the years.

The practitioners reading this may struggle with this characterization. If I refer back to the issues of ambivalence and prejudices, then I hope it is clear that I understand that some of this practitioner behaviour may stem from these. Disability awareness is not a mandatory part of practitioners' training. Moreover, childhood disability is not given much emphasis even where such awareness-raising does exist. Most people have to work this through for themselves, just as parents do. Clearly there are excellent examples of good practice where words such as 'partnership', 'relationship' and 'inclusion' have real meaning. It is important to acknowledge, though, how the lottery nature of these meetings – who you get, individual personalities, lack of clarity about roles and responsibilities – has a part to play in just how much of an emotional impact our particular parenting circumstances have on us and our families.

Men and women

Family life issues, including siblings, are explored in another chapter. Here I want to return to my earlier comments about the impact on parents in terms of their relationship with each other. The incidence of single parent households among families with a disabled child is disproportionately higher than the average.* This not only has

---

* McKay S, Atkinson A (2007) *Disability and Caring Among Families with Children: Family Employment and Poverty Characteristics.* Research Report No. 460. London: Department of Work and Pensions.

implications for the financial situation for those households, but also can be seen as an indicator of the stress on relationships when caring for one or more disabled children. Being parents is hard work and can prove challenging to the relationship itself. If a relationship is already struggling, then the extra care needs of a disabled child can lead to it breaking down.

Central to this is emotion – and how each person reacts and responds to their situation. While the additional needs of their baby or child can bring parents closer together, it is not unusual for each parent to react to their situation differently. Some of the feelings that can be around arise from a sense of loss and grief. Of course, not everyone experiences these feelings, and, rather significantly, within a relationship one parent might see any evidence of these feelings as a sort of betrayal of their child. Not every couple will feel positive about their child. Indeed it is possible to see that the positive outlook of one parent appears to generate a counter response of negativity in the other parent, and vice versa. By their very nature our emotions are often complex, contradictory and perplexing.

Jenni Thomas OBE refers to the very different ways that men and women grieve on the Child Bereavement Charity website (www.childbereavement.org.uk/understanding_ bereavement/how_men_and_women_grieve). She is speaking specifically about the loss of a child; however, much of this I find helpful when thinking about how men and women cope with being parents of a disabled child:

> Grief is solitary – even when other people around them are grieving, each parent can feel alone and normal patterns in their relationship may be disrupted. Couples often experience an inability to communicate feelings of grief to one another, to express the awfulness of their feelings.

She refers to women being more naturally loss-oriented and more concerned with their feelings. In contrast, men are more likely to be restoration-oriented. They want things to be repaired and to return to normal as soon as possible. These different ways of dealing with grief can put a significant strain on a relationship, and it is helpful for us to understand that each person's response to grief is natural. Once this is appreciated, it can become easier then to find ways of share feelings and reaching out to one another. Perhaps learning something from the other's approach can then help us to move on or to express something of what we are feeling. She also talks about how we can oscillate – move between the two. And how we can overlap, i.e. both be in restorative mode for a while – but that this can change again and itself be perplexing, even when we know what is going on.

In very general terms men and women can take on quite traditional roles when they become parents. Mothers become the main carer and fathers focus on providing for their family. In our modern society many women return to paid employment sometime after their child's birth and couples juggle the various demands of home, work and childcare between them. When a child has additional needs it can certainly feel as if there is less flexibility in terms of the options around employment. Indeed, parents of disabled children are three times more likely to be workless than other parents, with many parents having to take employment that fits their caring responsibilities rather than their skills and experience.* Men and women can then be forced into roles that do not fit with their personal or parental expectations, and this too can be a source of tension.

Fathers can, of course, be greatly affected emotionally by their child's disability, impairment or illness and tend to rely heavily on their partners for emotional support. The needs of fathers can be missed by services, which tend to focus on support for the child and mother. Going to work is a common coping strategy of fathers and important for identity and self-esteem. However, many fathers do not get the flexibility from employers and services that they need so that they can respond to their children's needs, such as attending appointments and being involved in the decisions and care relating to their child.

For many fathers the search for information can become a 'coping' strategy that works effectively for them for a while in helping them to come to terms with their child's condition. Knowledge is power, and so to understand what has occurred, what has 'caused' the difficulties and what 'might' happen as a result can be very empowering. However, as with the different forms of grieving the partner may not be able to 'hear' the information or experience the same enthusiasm for it. When you are in the midst of the feelings it can be very hard to understand what your partner is doing. Recognizing that the pursuit of information may be helpful for some fathers (and mothers) may help you to listen to what they say – or to state very clearly that you cannot but you are glad that it is helpful for them.

Joy and celebration

Clearly then the emotional impact for parents and families cannot be underestimated. Much of what I have explored has focused on what can be difficult and distressing, but of course joy, pleasure and delight have their part too. As every aspect of my son's development was delayed I began to move on from feeling sad at this to being thrilled at every bit of progress that he could make. 'Progress' can mean as much or as little as you make it. Adjusting your expectations will not always be easy. You will not always be able to make your child's only comparison point how he or she was six months ago, particularly once in school (mainstream or specialist), but, when you can, it can feel very good indeed.

Some parents report feeling that caring for their disabled child gives them a sense of purpose like no other, others that they constantly marvel at their child's ability to confront the challenges of life. Many more say that this is how he or she is and how loveable they are for all that!

---

* Lawton D (1998) *Complex Numbers: Families with More than One Disabled Child.* York: Social Policy Research Unit.

I would argue that for many of us it is easier to get to these feelings if we have been allowed and allowed ourselves to feel whatever else emerges. However, the context for this is support, emotional as well as practical.

Living with the life you have – acknowledging, adapting and adjusting

Even when our emotions are not particularly fierce or challenging to us, they can impact on how we feel about ourselves as parents, partners, lovers, friends, family and colleagues. This in turn impacts on our interactions with others, including our disabled child. It is natural to need acknowledgement from others for what we are feeling. At times we need to receive affirmation for our efforts and at others to be gently challenged.

We need those around us to understand this, and, in terms of the professionals involved with our families, adopt a proactive approach that acknowledges that our feelings can be complex. Many of us find it hard to ask for help, and if the messages from others appear to be that 'coping alone' and 'getting on with it' are virtuous behaviours then we are less likely to reach out for help. Being received by others without judgement and with compassion – not pity – can help us on the process of acknowledging, adapting and adjusting. Aspects of this process, I would argue, will be a regular feature for many of us throughout our child's life. Friends, family and the professionals involved with our children can help us through this process, but we may need to educate them to understand it and to recognize that they will be going through it at some level themselves.

Of course we have to get to that understanding ourselves, because without that the attitudes and responses of others will make little sense to us. It is important that we take care of ourselves and each other. Counselling does not appeal to everyone and is also not as widely available as it needs to be. However, my own experience of counselling helped me to safely express my feelings and to work through them. A few sessions of couple counselling helped my husband and me to better understand each other's grief processes. There can be financial implications of using counselling, but it may be money well spent if you find a skilled counsellor (information is available from the British Association of Counselling and Psychotherapy; www.bacp.org.uk).

Other than counselling and support groups, there are things that I have learned from my work with other parents that I know can be helpful. These are practical steps but are about helping us to recognize and manage our emotions. When we are in a meeting with a professional we generally do not want to be feeling vulnerable and weepy. We need to be able to hear what he or she is saying, state our own views and concerns, and talk together about how we can move forward. Although we need acknowledgement from the professionals of the emotional impact of what is happening to us, and sometimes of the task they are asking us to carry out with our child, we also need to be able to discuss our child's needs without collapsing into tears or becoming aggressive and defensive. When we know that an appointment is coming up, it can be helpful to talk through with a friend or family member what it is that we want from it. We need to be clear about our expectations and to write down questions and points that we really want to cover. However, I would argue that it is difficult to do this sometimes by ourselves, and so professionals working with us need to encourage us and offer their time to help us to prepare. Better use of a professional's time could on occasion be in helping us to talk through an impending meeting rather than carrying out some therapy treatment with our child. To recognize this, professionals really need to take on board the emotion associated for many of us with any meeting relating to our child's needs.

I have been very fortunate to receive a great deal of support from friends and colleagues. The therapeutic environment of my workplace (a voluntary organization supporting families of disabled children and young people) and regular practice supervision ensured that I came to a better understanding of my emotions and their impact on me and those around me. It is essential that those around us, working with us, have high self-awareness and can support us to come to terms with the emotional impact of being a parent of a disabled child. Personally, I feel better able to love and parent my son because I understand what I feel about him and the life I have because he is in it.

Summary
- Becoming a parent awakes many different emotions, and if that baby has difficulties and we are forced to adjust all our expectations, then these will include loss, grief, anxiety and anger.
- The society we live in is very ambivalent about disability, and this also colours our feelings towards our child. We need to acknowledge this in order to move on and accept our child for him or herself.
- We also need support and encouragement from those around us.
- Becoming a parent of a disabled child requires us to engage with a host of professionals and services. And these professionals also need to acknowledge and work through their own emotions.
- The baby's birth will also affect the parents' own relationship; the incidence of lone parent families with a disabled child is higher than average.
- Having a disabled child also tends to impose traditional roles on couples. Mothers become the main carer and fathers focus on providing for their family. As well as the financial impact, this can force people into roles that do not fit, which can be another source of tension.
- The emotional needs of fathers are often neglected; as they throw themselves into work they become less involved with their child's care. One 'coping mechanism' in trying to come to terms with their child's condition is searching for information.
- No matter how slow your child's progress, it will be cause for joy and celebration.

- In our process of adapting and adjusting to our new life, we all need acknowledgement of our feelings from those around us. Friends, family and the professionals involved with our children can help us through this process, but we may need to educate them to understand it.

- Counselling does not appeal to everyone, but it can help parents to safely express their feelings and to work through them, and couples to understand one another's grief processes. Support groups are also useful here.

- We need to prepare for meetings with professionals.

- The more aware we, and the people around us, are aware of how our emotions are woven into our life with our child, the better parents we can be to him or her.

About the author
Claire Edwards is the mother of Joe, who has Down syndrome with autistic features. She recently left her post as Director of SNIP (Special Needs Information Point, now KINDRED), a parent-led voluntary organization with bases in Edinburgh and Fife to become an independent trainer and consultant. She developed and still co-delivers SNIP's training programme for practitioners working with families of disabled children. She is currently the Chair of CCNUK (Care Coordination Network UK), a voluntary organization promoting care coordination and key working for families of disabled children and young people. She is a qualified counsellor but has not practised since the birth of her son in 2001, and in a previous life managed a large bookstore in Glasgow, moving up from London in 1988.

Useful resources
HemiHelp message board (www.board.hemihelp.org.uk): allows parents to share their concerns and experience.

Live Web Chat counselling service (www.scope.org.uk/Relate-live-web-chat-counselling-service): Scope has teamed up with trained Relate counsellors to deliver a live web chat service for families with disabled children.

Glossary of medical terms

Acquired Resulting from illness or injury after birth; not *congenital*.

Acute (medical) A short-lasting condition or illness (opposite of *chronic*).

Antidystonic Used to counteract *dystonia*.

Ascending pathway The system of *neurons* that carries information from our senses to our brain.

Basal ganglia Deep parts of the brain vital in the co-ordination and fluidity of movement.

Bilateral Affecting both sides.

Biomechanical Relating to the mechanics of the body: how the bones, muscles and tendons work together.

Brainstem Small part of the brain just above the spinal cord that relays motor and sensory information between the body and brain. It also regulates breathing, heart rate, temperature control and consciousness.

Central nervous system The brain and the spinal cord, through which messages pass between our brain and our muscles and senses.

Central pattern generators Networks of nerves that produce organized, rhythmic movements (like breathing and swallowing).

Cerebral To do with the brain.

Cerebral palsy See page 16.

Chronic (medical) A persistent, long-lasting or recurrent condition or injury (opposite of *acute*).

Clinical pathway, patient pathway, patient treatment pathway The route taken by a patient through all interactions with the health service.

Clonus Involuntary muscle twitching.

Cognition (adj Cognitive) Mental processes such as learning, remembering, understanding language, solving problems, and making decisions.

Congenital Developing or present before, at or very soon after around birth.

Contracture Shortening (of the muscle and tendon).

Contralateral On the opposite side.

Cortex Layers covering the *cerebral hemispheres*, responsible for our senses, thoughts, words and deeds.

Corticospinal, tract Main link between the cortex of the brain and the spinal cord, crossing over to interact with the other side of the body.

Descending (motor) pathway The system of *neurons* that takes messages from our brain to our muscles in order to control movement.

Dyskinesis See *Dystonia.*

Dystonia Loss of fluidity of motor control where sustained abnormal muscle contractions lead to involuntary movements (see also page 17).

Electroencephalography (EEG) An electrical recording of brain activity.

Equinus A walking position on tiptoes because the sole of the foot is permanently flexed downwards.

Flexion Bending (of a joint), being bent.

Growth plate The area of growing tissue at the end of a child's bone.

Haemorrhage Serious bleeding.

Hemiparesis See page 17.

Hemiplegia See page 17.

Hemisphere One of the two halves of the cerebrum (the largest part of the brain).

Hypertonia, spasticity Increased *muscle tone* or tightness (see also page 17).

Hypotonia Decreased *muscle tone*.

Intervention (medical) Treatment.

Intracranial Inside the skull.

Lesion Damage to a part of the body.

Locomotor driving system The part of the brain that manages the network of neurons controlling our muscles to produce movements.

Magnetic resonance imaging A technique used to obtain images of the inside of our body.

Motor (as in *motor control*) To do with movement.

Motor control The control of movements by the brain and nervous system.

Motor cortex The part of the *cortex* that controls movements.

Motor neuron, nerve A *neuron* that takes messages from the central nervous system to muscles.

Motor pathway The network of *motor neurons*.

Motor pattern generation The way in which nerves generate commands for muscles to carry out movements such as walking.

Motor unit A single *motor neuron* and the muscle fibres that it works with to produce movement.

MRI See *Magnetic resonance imaging*.

Muscle tone See *Tone*.

Neuron A nerve cell; helps carry messages and information to the brain and to and from the spinal cord.

Nervous system The network of brain, spinal cord and nerves that gets information from the body and sends it out to the body, controlling how we move, think, perceive and react, both consciously and subconsciously. Divided into the *central nervous system* and the *peripheral nervous system*.

Neural To do with the nervous system.

Neural pathways The connections between the different parts of the nervous system.

Neural plasticity, neuroplasticity The ability of the brain to adapt or 'rewire' after damage to compensate for the damage.

Neurology (adj. neurological) The study of the nervous system.

Occupational therapy Treatment aimed at making someone as independent as possible in their daily life, both by developing their skills and adapting their surroundings.

Ophthalmologist A doctor who treats eye problems.

Orthosis (pl orthoses) A splint.

Palsy Muscle stiffness or rigidity.

Pathway See *Motor pathway, Neural pathway, Clinical pathway*.

Patient pathway See *Clinical pathway*.

Patterning Use of repetitive movements or exercises.

Peripheral nervous system The network of neurons that carries messages to and from the *central nervous system*.

Periventricular Around a ventricle (e.g. in the brain).

Physiotherapy Treatment of muscles and joints using exercise and massage.

Plasticity See *Neural plasticity*.

Remodelling (of bone) Reshaping, forming of new bony tissue.

Secondary (disorder) Resulting from a primary or fundamental problem.

Spasticity See *Hypertonia*.

Tone (as in muscle tone) The natural state of partial contraction (tension or tightening) of a muscle.

Trauma (medical) Serious injury.

Glossary

Ultrasound A technique used to obtain images of the inside of our body.

Unilateral On one side.

Valgus Outward bending (of a joint).

Varus Inward bending (of a joint).

Vascular To do with blood vessels.

Ventricle (in the brain) One of four cavities in the brain.

Index

Index

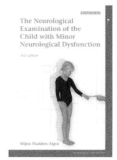

The Neurological Examination of the Child with Minor Neurological Dysfunction, 3rd edition

A practical guide from Mac Keith Press

Mijna Hadders-Algra

2010 • £49.95 • €60.00 • $72.00 • Paperback • 168 pp
ISBN 978-1-898683-98-8

This highly practical book brings the examination of minor neurological dysfunction developed by Bert Touwen and his colleagues in Groningen right up to date, which is timely in view of the increasing interest in and use of this approach. The approach is a detailed and extensive neurological examination with the aim of detecting a possible neurobiological basis for learning, behavioural and motor coordination problems in a child and thus informing decision-making and management. It provides a refined, sensitive and age-appropriate technique, designed to take into account the developmental aspects of the child's rapidly changing nervous system.

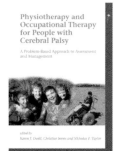

Physiotherapy and Occupational Therapy for People with Cerebral Palsy: a problem-based approach to assessment and management

A practical guide from Mac Keith Press

Edited by Karen J. Dodd, Christine Imms and Nicholas F. Taylor

2010 • £29.95 • €35.90 • $39.99 • Paperback • 256 pp
ISBN 978-1-898683-68-1

This book is a practical resource for physiotherapists and occupational therapists who support people with cerebral palsy, helping them to solve the problems with movement and other impairments that so often accompany cerebral palsy, so that they can be more active and better able to participate in roles such as study, work, recreation and relationships.

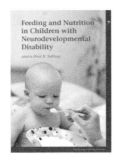

Feeding and Nutrition in Children with Neurodevelopmental Disability

A practical guide from Mac Keith Press

Edited by Peter B. Sullivan

2009 • £20.00 • €24.00 • $40.00 • Paperback 196 pp
ISBN 978-1-898683-60-5

This book is for all those who have responsibility for the nutritional and gastrointestinal care of children with neurodisability, providing an up-to-date account of the practicalities of assessment and management of feeding problems in these children. The emphasis throughout is on the importance of team-based care: it is written from a multidisciplinary perspective by a group of authors with considerable clinical and research experience in this area.

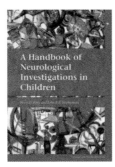

A Handbook of Neurological Investigations in Children

A practical guide from Mac Keith Press

Mary D. King and John B.P. Stephenson

2009 • £39.95 • €46.00 • $69.95 • Paperback • 399 pp
ISBN 978-1-898683-69-8

The number of possible neurological investigations is now very large indeed, and uncritical investigations may be seriously misleading and often costly. In this book the authors set out the investigations that are really needed to establish the cause of neurological disorders in children. Their problem-oriented approach starts with the patient's presentation, not the diagnosis. More than 60 case vignettes of real children illustrate clinical scenarios.

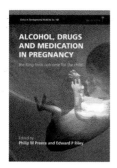

**Alcohol, Drugs and Medication in Pregnancy:
the long-term outcome for the child**

Edited by Philip M. Preece and Edward P. Riley

Clinics in Developmental Medicine No. 188
2011 • £65.00 • €78.00 • $95.00 • Hardback • 256 pp
ISBN 978-1-898683-88-9

This book documents the outcome and consequences for children
exposed to intrauterine drugs, alcohol and medicines. In setting out
the evidence for these outcomes, the authors demonstrate that
decisions about future care and management can and should be
made early, with a secure understanding of the effect of this early
exposure. This should allow professionals to provide protective
management and prevent the delays in intervention and decision
making that have so often been seen in this area of medical and
social care.

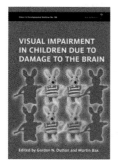

Visual Impairment in Children due to Damage to the Brain

Edited by Gordon N. Dutton and Martin Bax

Clinics in Developmental Medicine No. 186
2010 • £80.00 • $135.00 • €96.00 • Hardback • 224 pp
ISBN 978-1-898683-86-5

This ambitious book links the work of authors from many of the
major research teams in this field, who have made significant
contributions to the literature on the subject of cerebral visual
impairment and provides a structured amalgam of the viewpoints
of different specialists. The book contains some very novel
concepts, which will be of great practical value to those who care
for children with visual impairment due to brain injury.

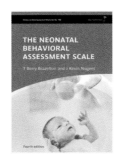

The Neonatal Behavioral Assessment Scale, 4th edition

T. Berry Brazelton and J. Kevin Nugent

Clinics in Developmental Medicine No. 190
2011 • £50.00 • €60.00 • $63.95 • Hardback • 200 pp
ISBN 978-1-907655-03-6

The Neonatal Behavioral Assessment Scale (NBAS) is the most comprehensive examination of newborn behaviour available today and has been used in clinical and research settings around the world for more than 35 years. The scale assesses the newborn's behavioral repertoire with 28 behavioral items and also includes an assessment of the infant's neurological status on 20 items

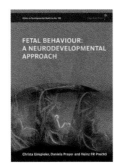

Fetal Behaviour: A Neurodevelopmental Approach

Christa Einspieler, Daniela Prayer and Heinz FR Prechtl

Clinics in Developmental Medicine No. 189
2011 • £70.00 • €84.00 • $109.95 • Hardback • 176 pp
ISBN 978-1-898683-87-2

Fetal behaviour and movements not only give an insight into the developing brain, as an expression of neural activity, but are also necessary for the further development of neural structure and of other organs. This book presents an account of our current understanding of fetal behaviour as obtained through the assessment of fetal movements and behavioural states. The approach is based on the premises of developmental neurology, and provides important clues for the recognition of the age-specific functional repertoire of the nervous system. The companion DVD contains 26 movies using both ultrasound and dynamic MRI to illustrate the text.